# *Medieval Crafts*
## *a book of days*

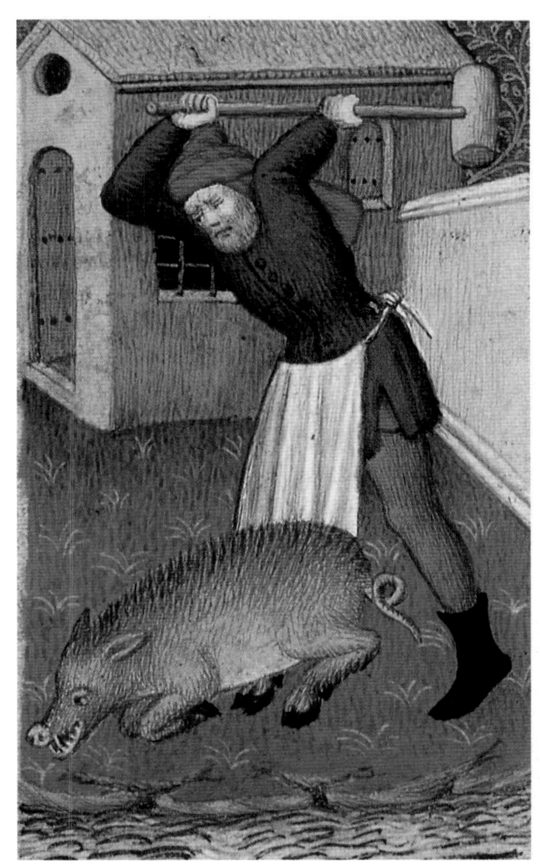

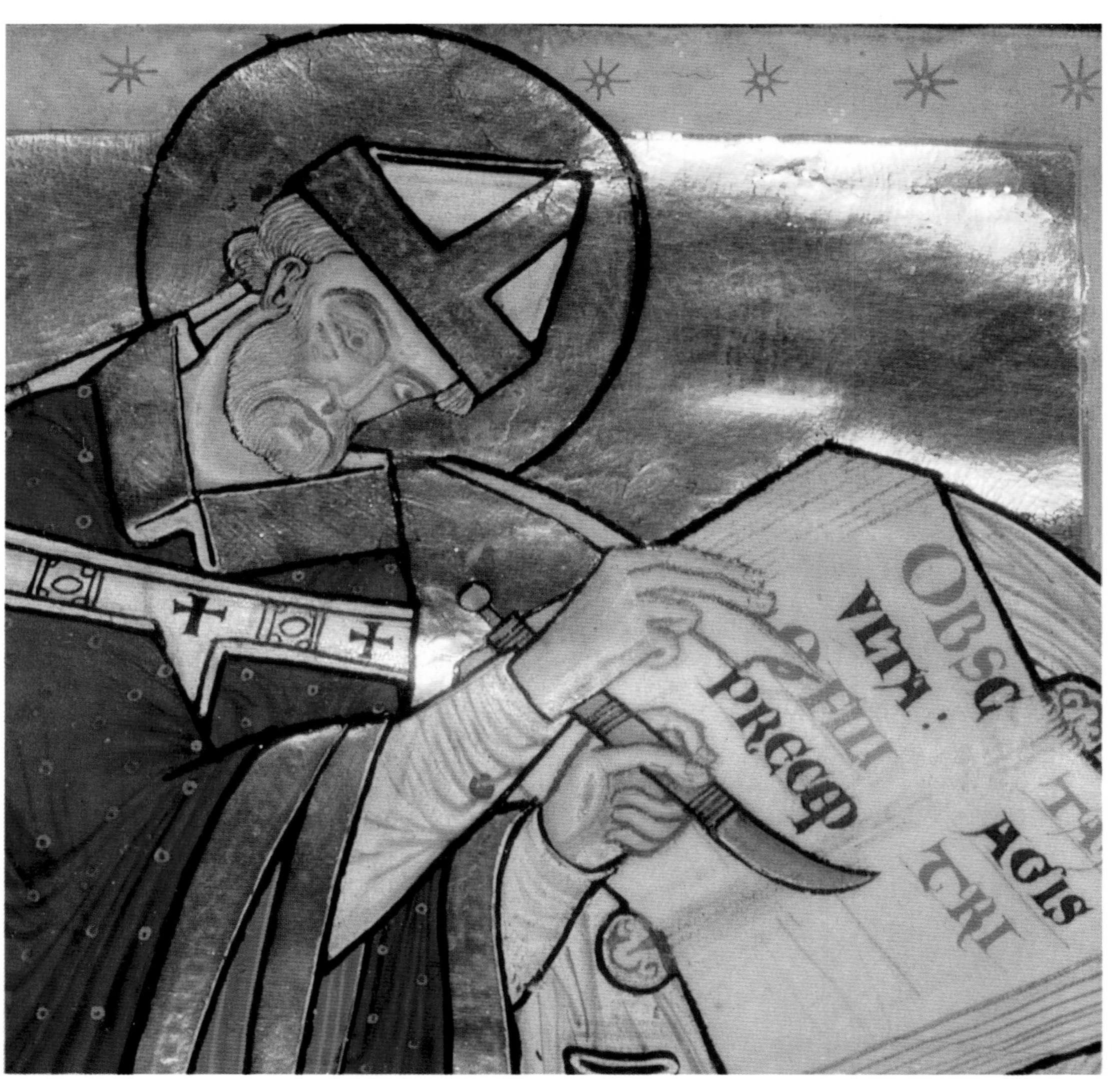
OBSC
VLTA:
PRECEP
AGIS
TRI

# Medieval Crafts

## a book of days

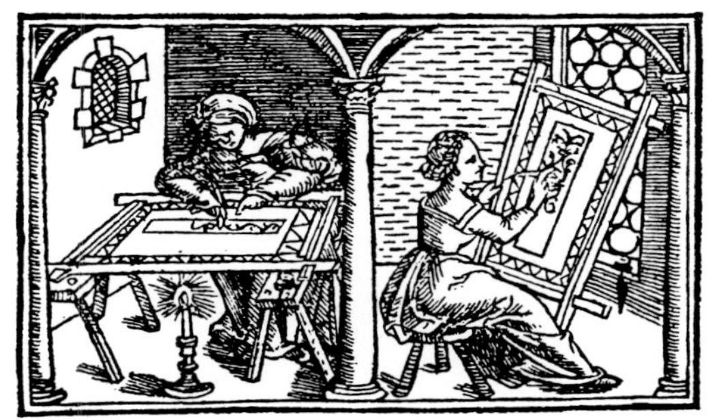

JOHN CHERRY

THAMES AND HUDSON

*Cover* The German minstrel Hartman von Starkenberg forging a helmet.

*Back cover* Masons using a scaffolding platform and completing a tower from inside.

*Half title* The Labour of the Month for December often shows a boar being killed. Fifteenth century.

*Title page left* St Dunstan copies a manuscript of the Rule of St Benedict. This illumination of *c.* 1170 shows him writing big coloured initials with a pen, while he holds down his parchment with a curved penknife. *Right* Woman transferring embroidery designs by pricking and pouncing, from a pattern book of 1527.

*Right* St Peter and other apostles hear the command of Christ. English embroidery of 1315–35 on an altar frontal showing scenes from the Passion of Christ.

*Far right* A design for tiles in Carew Cheriton Church, Dyfed.

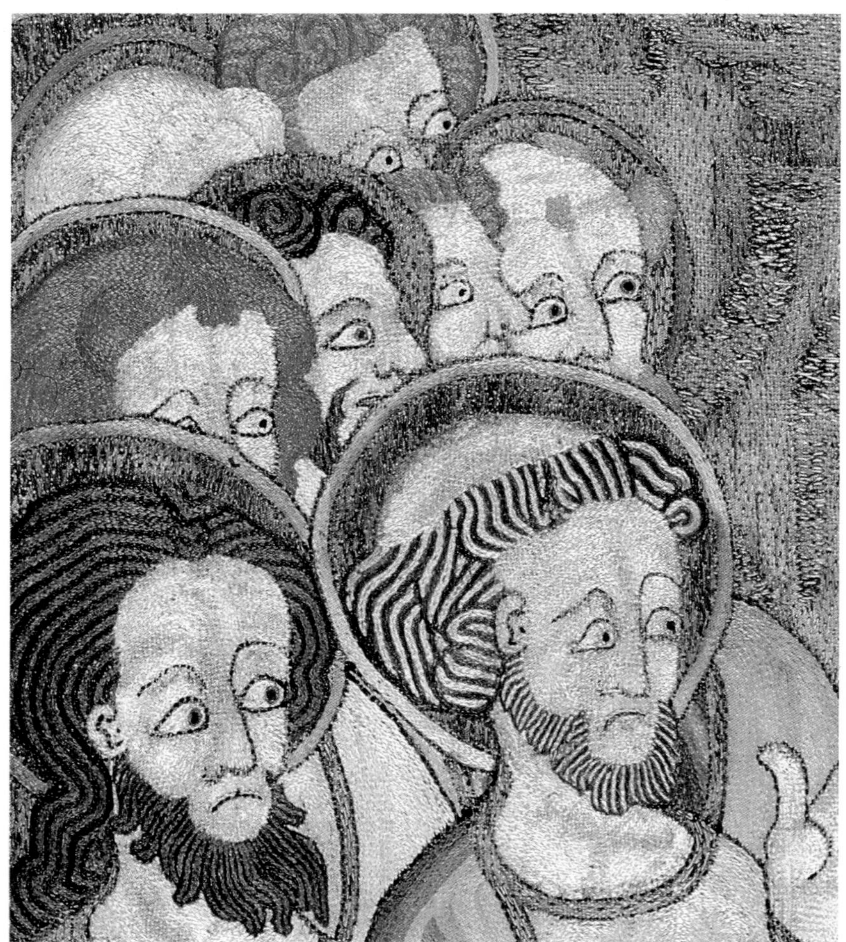



**First published in the United States of America in 1993 by Thames and Hudson Inc., 500 Fifth Avenue, New York, New York 10110**

**Published by arrangement with British Museum Press**



**Designed by Roger Davies**

**Printed in Italy**

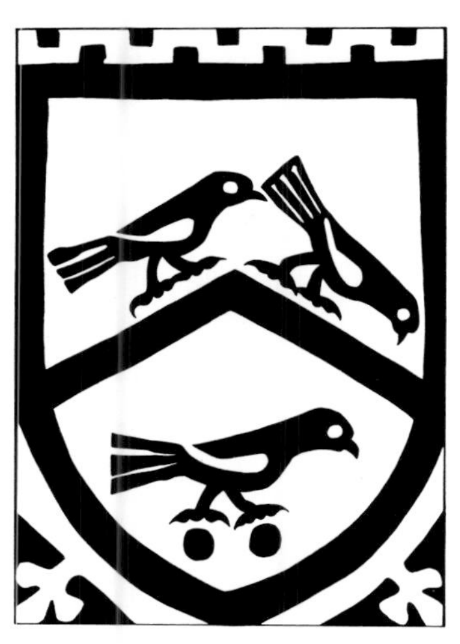

# Contents

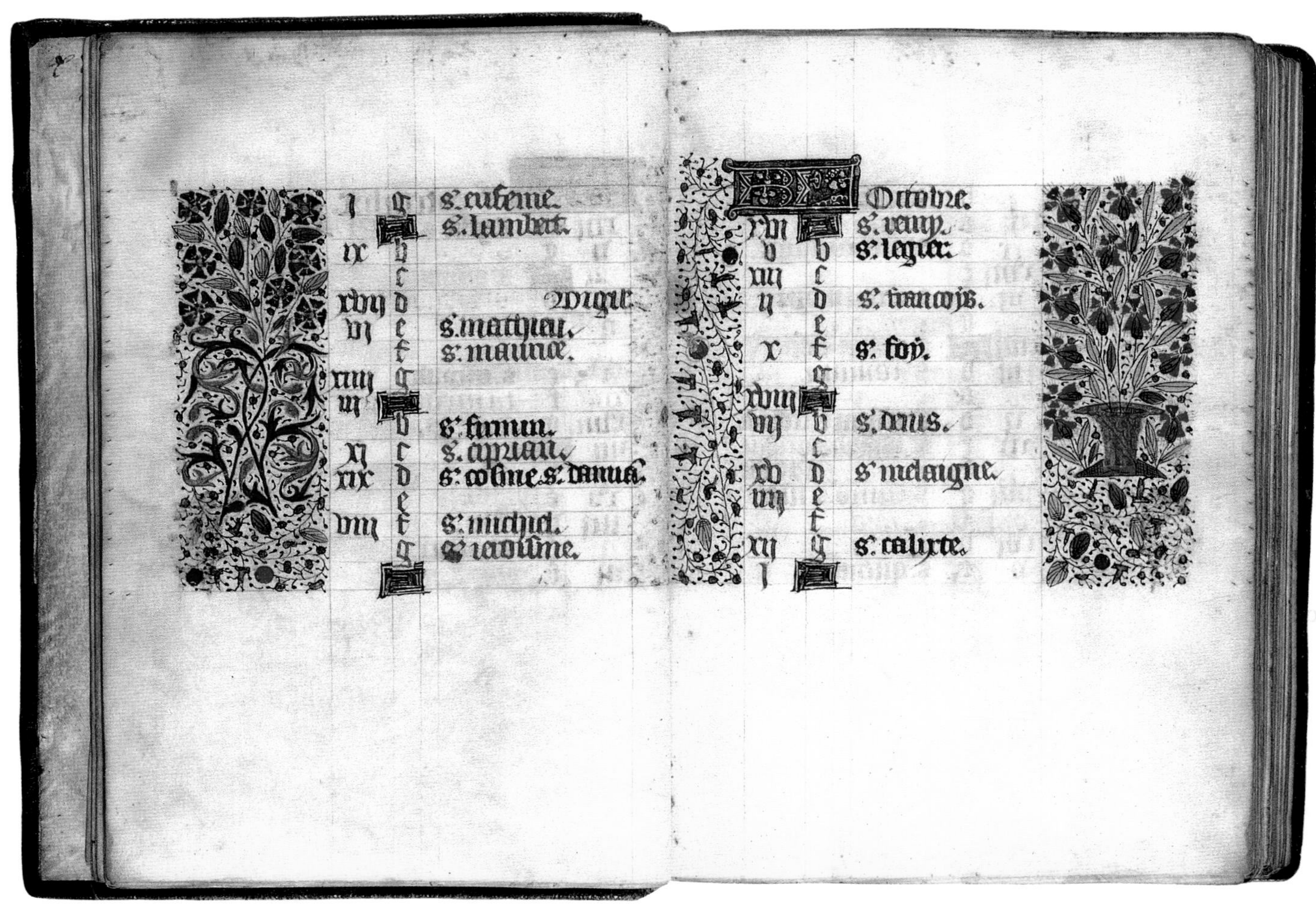

*Above* This calendar for September and October from a Book of Hours shows the principal saints' days in burnished gold, while the other names are in red and blue ink.

*Right above* God, as architect of the universe, creates the world with a giant pair of compasses. From the fourteenth-century Holkham Bible Picture Book.

# Introduction

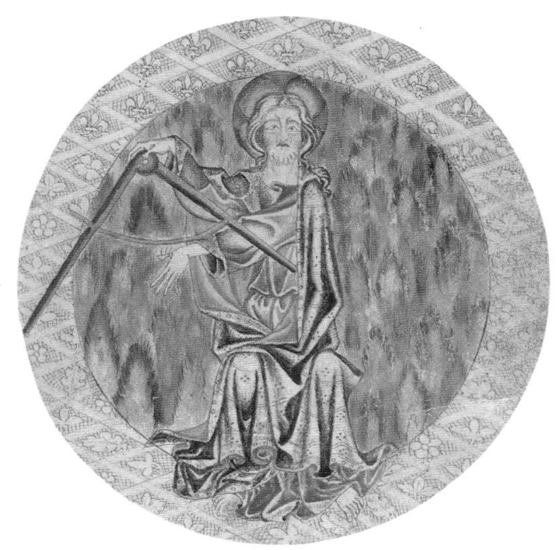

PAST TIMES communicate their character through their craftsmanship. Our first impression of the Middle Ages is sometimes the inside of a church decorated with its stained glass and stone sculpture, sometimes the outside of a castle with its towers and battlements, sometimes the gleam of gold and enamel in a museum showcase. The purpose of this Book of Days is to give an impression of some of the crafts and the craftsmen whose work can still give joy and understanding to us so long after its creation.

A craft was, and still is, the exercise of a manual skill which creates artefacts from a raw material. The crafts considered here are not those concerned with the production of raw material, such as mining or forestry or the operation of agriculture and fishing, but those which concern the production of an end product, often of great artistic quality, from the raw material. An element of fine art and creative design entered into all the crafts considered here. Some of the craftsmen have left permanent memorials such as buildings, stained glass windows and suits of armour, whilst others, particularly the cooks, have, by the very nature of their product, left nothing. Since this Book of Days records the passage of time, let us consider time in the Middle Ages and, in particular, how medieval craftsmen spent their days. What did time mean to the medieval craftsmen?

The passing of time in the Middle Ages was marked by the ringing of bells rather than the ticking of clocks. Bells were rung for both religious and secular occasions. Bells were rung for the daily services of the church. In monasteries, different methods of ringing distinguished each particular service in the monastic day. Bells were rung at the great church festivals, such as Christmas and Easter, as well as on the festivals of particular saints. A custom which had both an ecclesiastical and a secular character was the ringing of the Ave Bells, at the time when people rose and when they retired to bed, in order to remind them to say their prayers. In 1399 Archbishop Arundel ordered that the custom of saluting the Virgin Mary at daybreak and at curfew be universally adopted in the province of Canterbury, and that the bell to be rung was to be called the Gabriel Bell in memory of the Salutation of Our Lady, '*Ave Maria Gratia Plena*' (Hail Mary, Full of Grace). Bells were also rung for the opening and closing of markets, for the summoning of meetings, and for recalling scholars to their colleges. Occasionally bells were used to summon and dismiss workmen. In 1532, for instance, a frame was made for a bell in the White Tower in the Tower of London 'the whiche callith workemen to worke and fro worke'. Finally, bells were rung both before death to mark the passing of the soul, so that others could pray for the soul of the deceased, and at funerals, which represented the passing of the body into the grave. The rich goldsmith, Sir Martin Bowes, in his will of 1578 provided for forty pounds to be distributed to the poor 'on the day that he shall be in peril of death, whilst yet he still be alive and before the bell toll for him'. The craft of bell founding is illustrated by a stained glass window in York Minster, the Bellfounder's window in the north nave aisle, paid for by Richard Tunnoc, a bell founder and Mayor of York, who died in 1330.

One of the great contrasts between crafts in the Middle Ages and later methods of production is that the medieval craftsmen produced their work in daylight. It was clearly possible for them to work at night by using artificial light such as lanterns, torches, or candles, but it was quite rightly thought that the best work could only be performed in full daylight. Since craftsmen often sold their own products either in their workshops or in shops next door, an intending purchaser could be cheated if the light was poor. The regulations for working at night varied from craft to craft depending on the technical finesse required. It was often assumed that much incompetent and sometimes deceitful work went on at night. According to the London spur makers in 1345 'no man can work so neatly at night as by day and many people engaging in deceitful work prefer to do so by night'. The London smiths banned night work in 1296 and the London cutlers did the same in 1344. This emphasis on the use of daylight led naturally to a seasonal division of the working year.

Many crafts divided the year into a long summer and a short winter. In the fourteenth century, London blacksmiths apparently worked from 6 a.m. to 8 p.m. between November and January, and from dawn until 9 p.m. throughout the rest of the year. Such hours in the winter would hardly have been possible without artificial light. The building trade in Beverley in Yorkshire provides documentary evidence for the timetable of the working day in the fifteenth century. In summer, that is from Easter until 15 August, there was work from 4 to 6 a.m., 6.15 to 8 a.m., 8.30 to 11 a.m. when there was a one and a half hour break. Work resumed at 12.30 to 3 p.m. and from 3.30 to 7 p.m. In winter, work was from dawn to dusk, with breakfast from 9 to 9.30 a.m., dinner from midday to 1 p.m., and a break for a quarter of an hour at 3 p.m. The times in Beverley fit quite well with the Act of Parliament passed in 1495 which fixed the summer

*Right* The craft of bell founding; *left*, the turning of the bell and *right*, the casting of the bell. From the early fourteenth-century stained glass window given by Richard Tunnoc in the north aisle of York Minster.

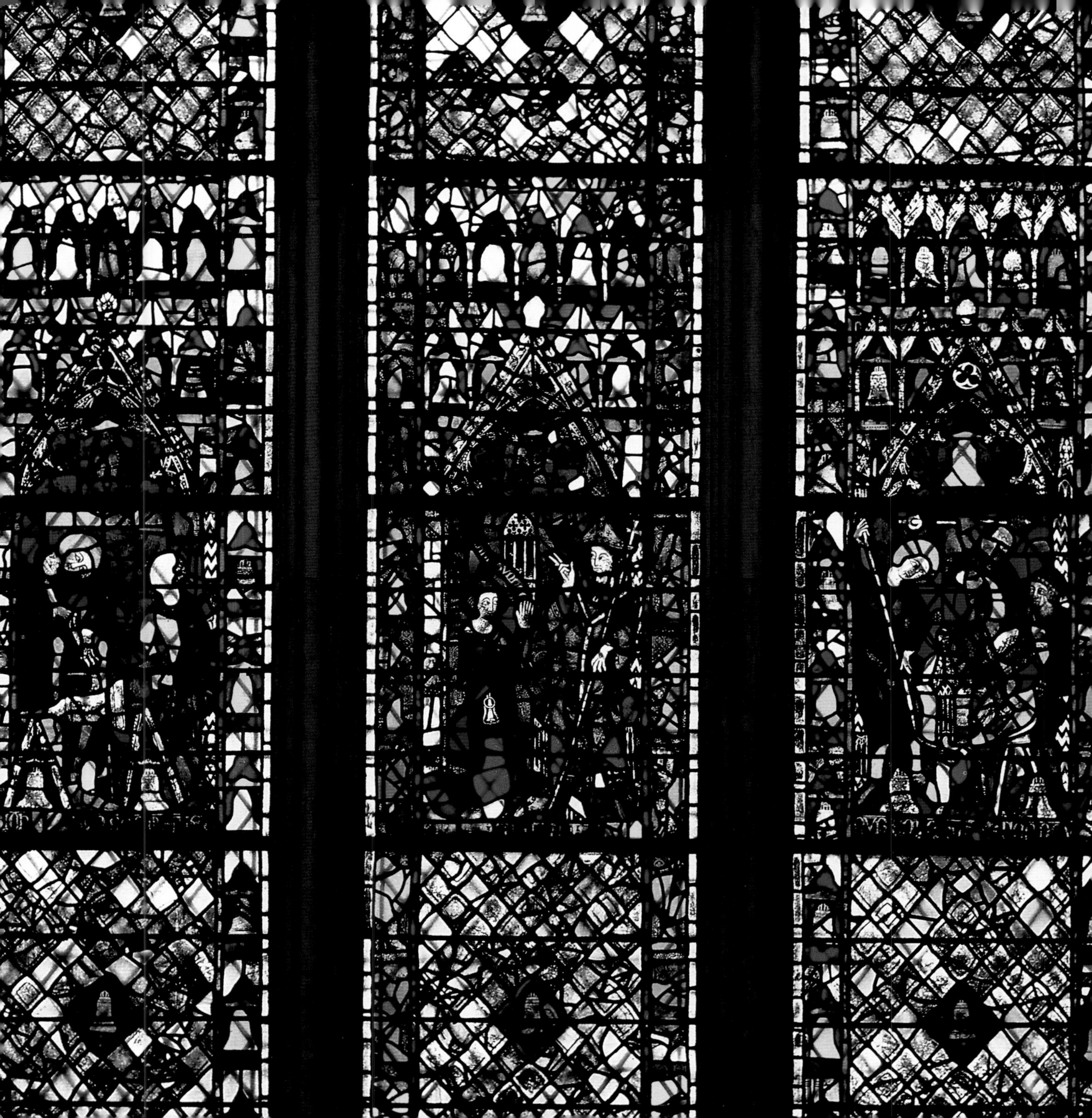

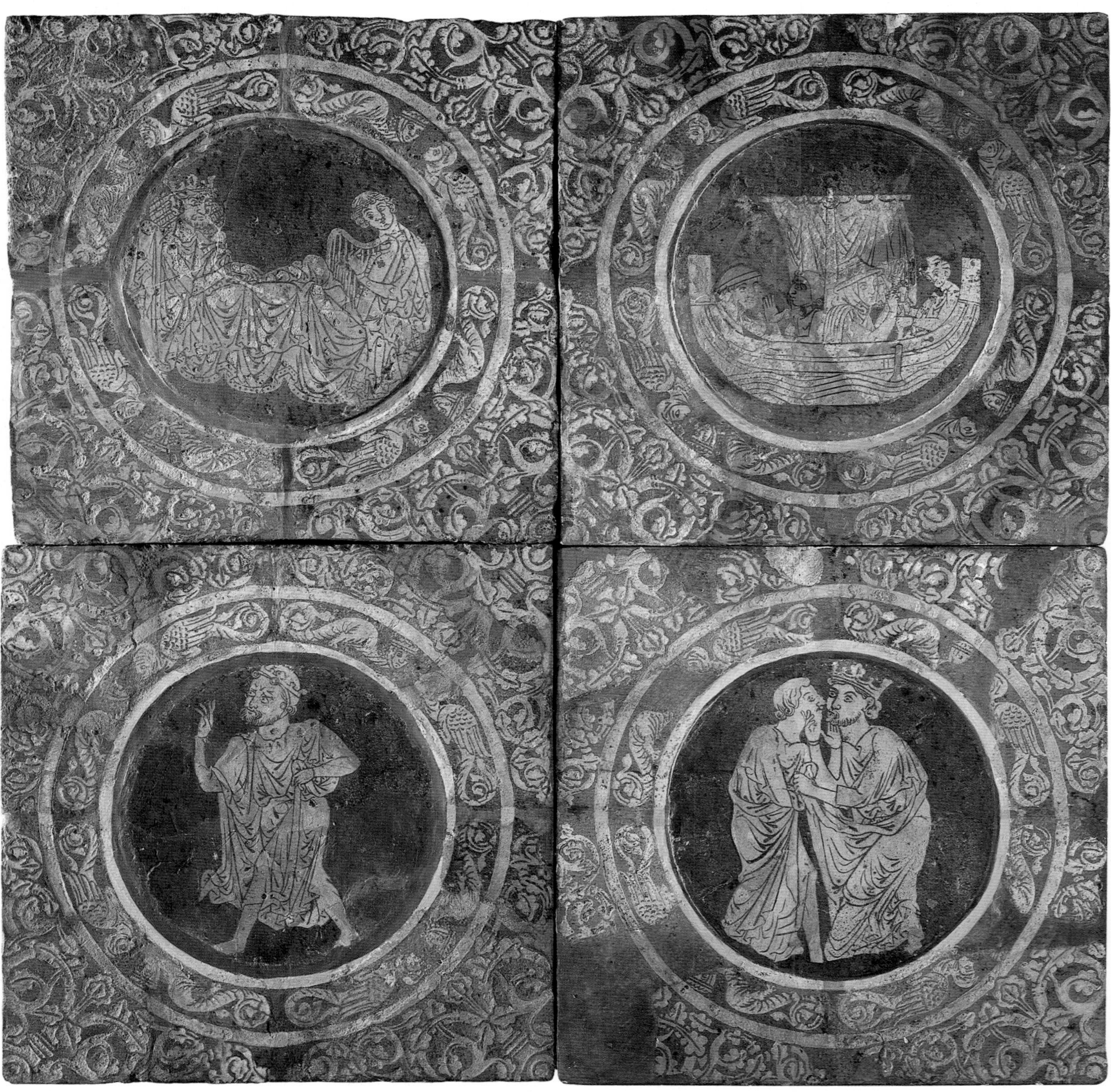

hours, from mid-March to mid-September, from 5 a.m. to between 7 and 8 p.m. with half an hour for breakfast and an hour and a half for dinner and sleep, and the winter hours from 'the springing of the day' until nightfall. The distinction between the summer and winter periods varied in different places. In London, the year was divided at Easter and Michaelmas (29 September), in Bristol, at Ash Wednesday and the Feast of St Calixtus (14 October) and, in the case of the workmen at Westminster, at the Purification of Our Lady (2 February) and All Saints' Day (1 November). The wages paid to workmen differed between winter and summer, according to the length of the day worked. The craftsman clearly deserved his money for the very long days worked in the summer.

Against the long hours worked we have to set the frequency of holidays. No work was done on Sundays and on all the great Church festivals, as well as on a number of local festivals. On Saturdays or on the day preceding the festival work ceased either at noon or sometimes at four o'clock. In the case of the bronze founders of London, while ordinary metalworking was not allowed after noon had been rung on a Saturday, they were permitted to complete a casting that was in progress. No one was allowed to work on Sundays, with the exception of farriers who, in Coventry at least, were expected to shoe the horses of travellers passing through the town. The Sunday opening of shops, then as now, presented problems. In the case of the London pastelers or restaurant keepers, only one shop in Bread Street and one in Bridge Street might be open on Sundays, the others being closed so that the staff might 'serve Godde the better on the Sonday as trew Cristen men shuld do'.

Some medieval craft work was seasonal, particularly where outdoor work was influenced by the weather. One of the most obvious examples of such seasonal work was the making of floor and roof tiles. In this process clay was dug in the fields in Autumn (before 1 November) and carted to the yard, where it was left in heaps until Christmas, then turned over (before 1 February) and left until Spring. The frost and rain broke up the clay and it was easier to work. The tilers would form their tiles in April and May in an open-fronted shed containing long forming tables. The tiles were then dried and fired in kilns, the firing of the kilns usually taking place between June and August. Another craft susceptible to weather and hence to the seasons was that of the masons and sculptors. In theory, building ceased from Michaelmas (29 September) until Easter, but in practice it ceased from All Saints' Day (1 November) until the Purification of the Virgin (2 February). Unfinished masonry had to be protected by a covering of turf, heather, or tiles. This was not always carried out and it was the absence of such protection in the early thirteenth century that caused the west front of the church of St Albans to crumble into ruin.

If we turn to the life of the craftsman it is clear that it was sometimes a great help to be born into the right family. In Augsburg, for instance, the sons of master armourers were exempt from both the years of apprenticeship and work as a journeyman. However, not all crafts required apprenticeships. Those that did were the trades where the guild organisation was strong. The period of apprenticeship varied with each craft. By the middle of the fourteenth century it

*Left* Tiles showing scenes from the romance of Tristram and Isolde. Made by tilers at Chertsey Abbey between 1260 and 1280.

was a general rule that entry to a London craft guild should be by an apprenticeship of not less than seven years. It was widely accepted that the best age at which to begin was 13 or 14 years so that the period of training may have been completed by the age of 20 or 21. Apprenticeship as such is not recorded until the reign of Edward I (1272–1307) and before that training was probably in the family, or on a more informal basis.

The amount of time it took for a craftsman to complete his work varied considerably. Some medieval cathedrals, like Cologne, were never completed. Some major pieces of goldsmith's work, such as shrines, also took years to complete. In 1292, the chapter of Beverley Minster in Yorkshire drew up a contract with the goldsmith, Roger of Faringdon, for a new shrine for the relics of their saint, John of Beverley, but for reasons unknown to us the shrine was not finished until 1308. In contrast, on some occasions work had to be produced in a great hurry. An order was given on 8 September 1352 to the French 'armeurier au Roy et brodeur', Nicolas Waquier, for a horse covering and room-hanging of velvet ornamented with 8,544 embroidered fleurs-de-lis to be completed by All Saints' Day. The embroidery work went on day and night and was only achieved by the provision of candles and wine. Sometimes, after they had completed their task, the craftsmen had to wait a considerable time before their bills were paid. Thomas Frowyk, a London goldsmith, was commissioned to make a crown for Margaret, the second Queen of Edward I, in 1303. When he subsequently applied for payment he was sent from one department of the royal administration to another before eventually receiving his money in stages. Clearly the craftsman was sometimes sorely tried by bureaucracy.

At the end of his life the successful craftsman and prominent member of his guild would expect a suitable funeral. Some set aside sums of money in their wills so that they should be remembered. In addition to the forty pounds for the poor already mentioned, Sir Martin Bowes left the sum of £13. 6s. 8d. to the wardens and commonalty of the goldsmiths to pay for an honest dinner for them at Goldsmiths' Hall on the day of his burial. Such prominent craftsmen were often anxious that their funerals were well attended and Bowes also left another payment to encourage twenty parish clerks to attend the funeral. The Ordinances of the Goldsmiths' Company of London stated that when anyone who was of the livery or fellowship of the Company died, every member of the livery of the craft should be present at his funeral. This was often stressed in wills such as that of Humphrey Coke, chief carpenter to Henry VIII, who, in 1531, desired 'that my crafte and occupacion of carpynters and all other brotherhoodes as I am of shall be at my burying'.

Many of the craft guilds had particular saints as their patrons. The armourers looked to St George (feast day 23 April), who was a military saint, while the painters were devoted to St Luke (18 October). He was supposed to have portrayed the Virgin Mary in the flesh, and is sometimes represented as a painter with his pots and brushes. The scribes and illuminators, however, favoured St John the Baptist (29 August). The feast day of the patron saint was usually an opportunity for celebration and for the annual meeting of the guild at which new wardens or officers were elected and the necessary business transacted. St Dunstan's Day (15 May), for example, was the principal ceremonial day for the London goldsmiths. It was marked by a special bell ringing at St Paul's Cathedral at the craft's expense. All the goldsmiths' shops were shut, the whole Company assembled in full livery, the new wardens were installed and the day

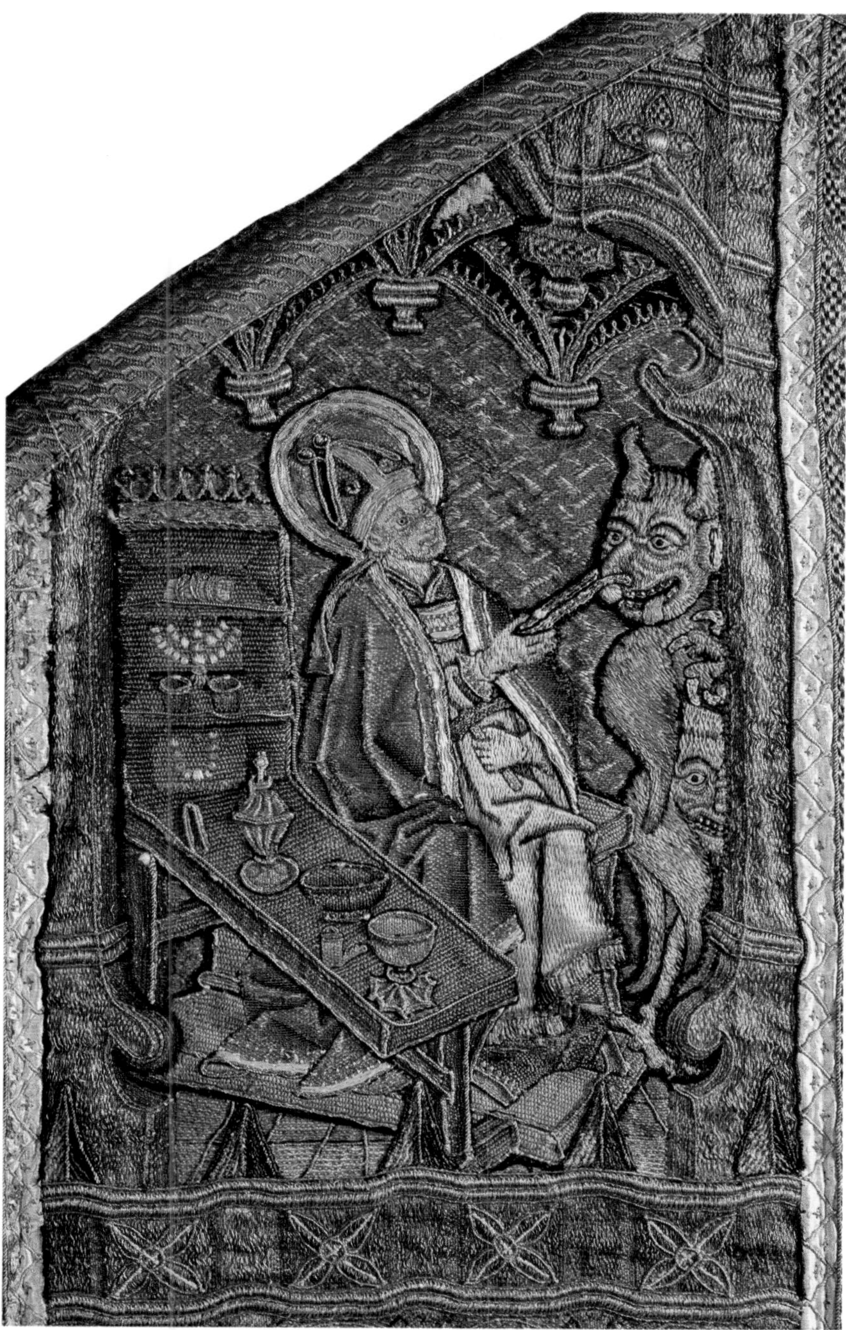

This scene on the Stonyhurst Chasuble is an example of *opus anglicanum* embroidery using silk, gold and silver thread on velvet. It was produced *c.* 1470. It shows St Dunstan, the patron saint of goldsmiths, in his workshop. He tweaks, with his goldsmiths' pliers, the nose of the monstrous devil who has interrupted his work. In the cupboard are displayed rings and rosary beads, while on his bench there are a mazer and a covered cup with spiral decoration.

was rounded off with a feast that was attended by all members of the Company. The feast given by the wardens to their predecessors in 1497 is recorded in some detail. There were three courses. The first consisted of four dishes: venison, roast capon, pike and baked venison; the second comprised cream of almonds, rabbit with chicken, turbot, pigeon and tarts, and the third strawberries and cream. At the St Dunstan's Day entertainment the following year, thirty-two gallons of red wine, eight gallons of claret and two barrels of ale were consumed. For other feasts payments to minstrels are recorded and it is clear that these events, marking the passing of the year in the history of the guild, were lavish occasions of considerable merriment.

The medieval craftsman sometimes depicted the passing of time. One way in which he did so was to represent the Labours of the Months. These may be found in the calendars of illuminated manuscripts, on the portals of cathedrals, in wall paintings and on the tiles that decorated floors. The symbols used for the different months were based on a much-repeated tradition. Some of the more interesting scenes may be noted here, though none, alas, show craftsmen at work. January is often illustrated by a man with two heads representing youth and age; one face looks back to the past while the other looks forward to the future. February shows the peasant at home warming himself in front of the fire. The series at Chartres and Sens Cathedrals show the peasant trimming his vines in March. April was thought to be the most beautiful month in the Middle Ages. With its bright sunshine and capricious nature, it is portrayed as a youth crowned with flowers. May shows the knight hawking or hunting. June is the month for mowing meadows. In July the peasant cuts the corn with a sickle, and the harvest is threshed with a flail in August. In France, September is often shown as the month when the grapes are gathered in for the vintage. The sowing of the seed by the peasant, scattering it with a sweep of his arm, usually represents October. November is the time to prepare for winter and the peasant is depicted chopping wood or fattening his pigs on the acorns blown down by the autumn winds in readiness for the December feasts. December is a time for rest, rejoicing and repasts, represented by activities such as the killing of pigs and the baking of cakes. Sometimes December is shown feasting with a glass before him. The scenes that the craftsmen depicted were essentially those of the agricultural year. Secure within his sculptor's lodge or illuminator's workroom, the craftsman portrayed the cultivator of the land as he stood, frequently alone, in his conflict with nature.

Among the many decorative programmes that Henry III ordered for his royal palaces, time had its part. The fireplace in the Queen's Hall at Clarendon was rebuilt in 1250 with marble columns on either side and carved with the symbols of the twelve months. He also ordered a decorated mantel at Westminster painted with 'a figure of Winter which by its sad countenance and by other miserable contortions of the body may be likened to Winter itself.'

These have all gone. Subjected to the decay and destruction of time, they are no more. However, some of the work of the medieval craftsmen still survives and can be seen today in castles, churches and museums. In this respect, the medieval craftsman lives on and has cheated time through the survival of his craft.

*Right* A man with a long pole knocks down ripe acorns to feed the pigs below. This fine example of the wood carvers' art on an early fourteenth-century gittern provides an example of the scene that often represents the month of November.

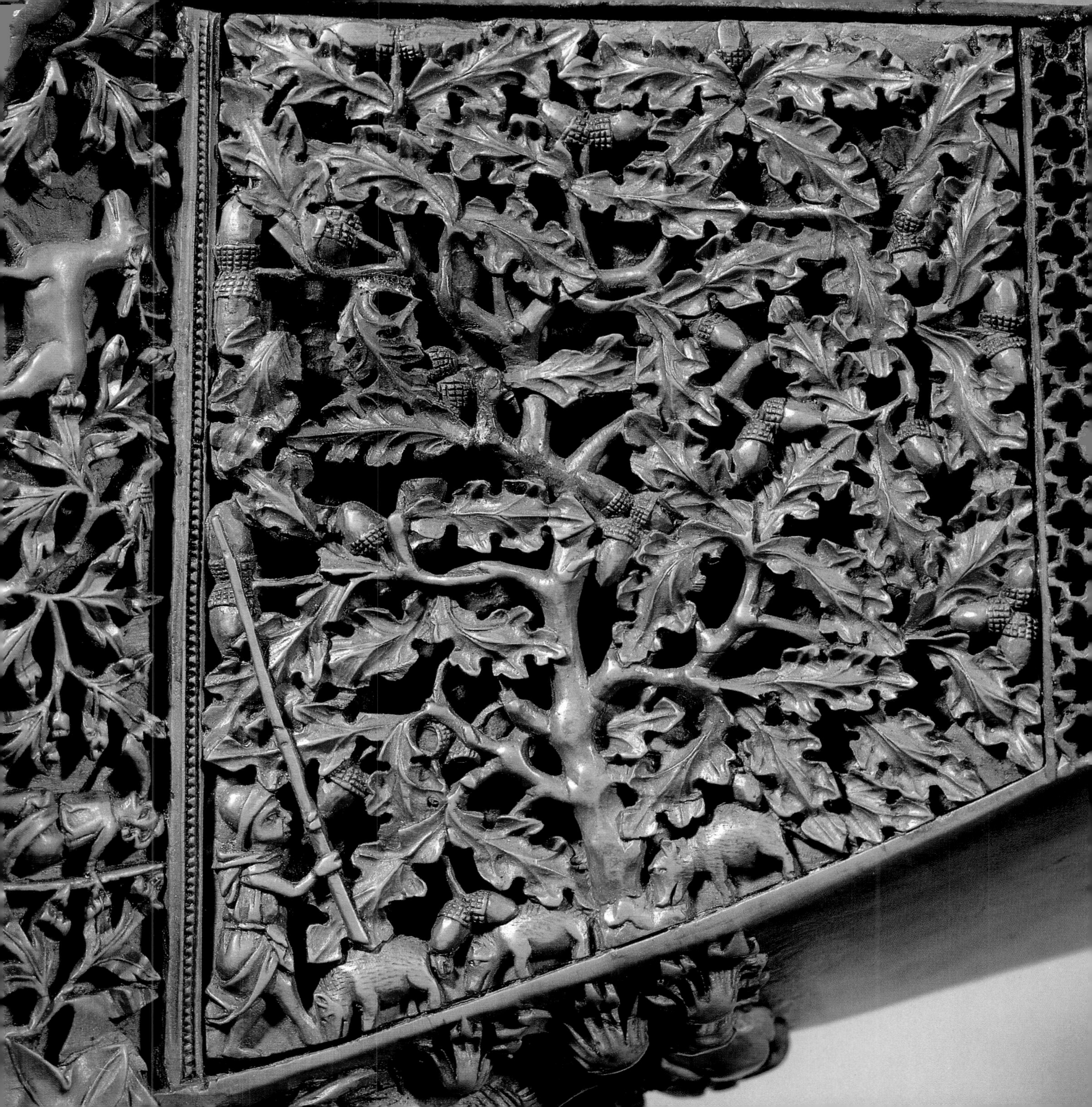

# January

SCRIBES

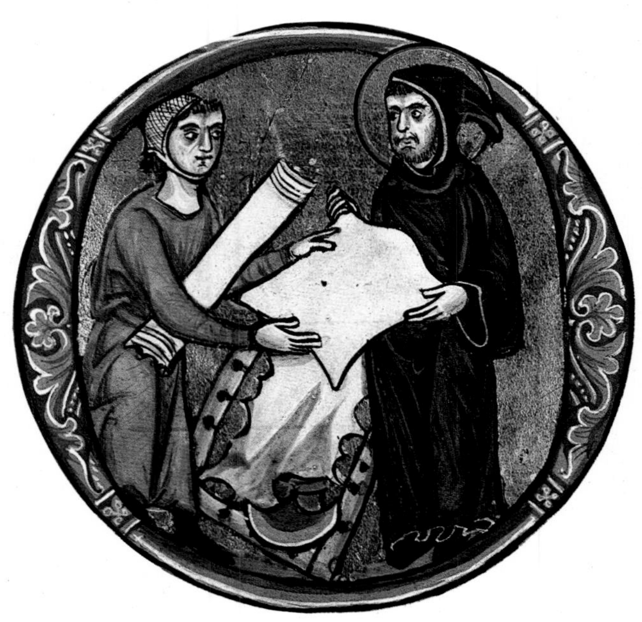

UNTIL ABOUT 1100 most manuscripts were copied by monks for use in monastic libraries. The increase in the number of new texts at that time led monasteries to employ secular scribes to produce books to keep their libraries up to date. The expansion of universities in the twelfth century resulted in increased book production and by 1200 secular workshops were writing and decorating manuscripts for sale to the laity. By 1300 it was exceptional for monasteries to make their own manuscripts.

Scribes would write on parchment or vellum. The preparation of parchment is a long and complicated process but the end result is an extraordinarily durable product. Paper made from linen rags was produced in France by about 1340, and in Germany by 1390, but probably not in England until the late fifteenth century. The scribe wrote with quill pens which frequently needed sharpening. In the twelfth century it was reported that a clerk taking dictation would need to sharpen his pen so often that he had to have sixty quills ready and sharpened in advance.

Some 19,000 signatures of medieval scribes in colophons of medieval manuscripts have been recorded, which means that scribes were perhaps the least anonymous of our craftsmen. Some simply give the name, such as Rogerius or Johannes. Many were women.

There were a great variety of scribes, ranging from clerks, students, priests and debtors to book owners themselves. The most amusing colophons are those in which a scribe declares his delight in finishing the task, often complaining of its length and asking for eternal life, a jug of wine, or a pretty girl in reward.

*Left* A parchment maker shows his product to a monk. From a thirteenth-century French manuscript initial.

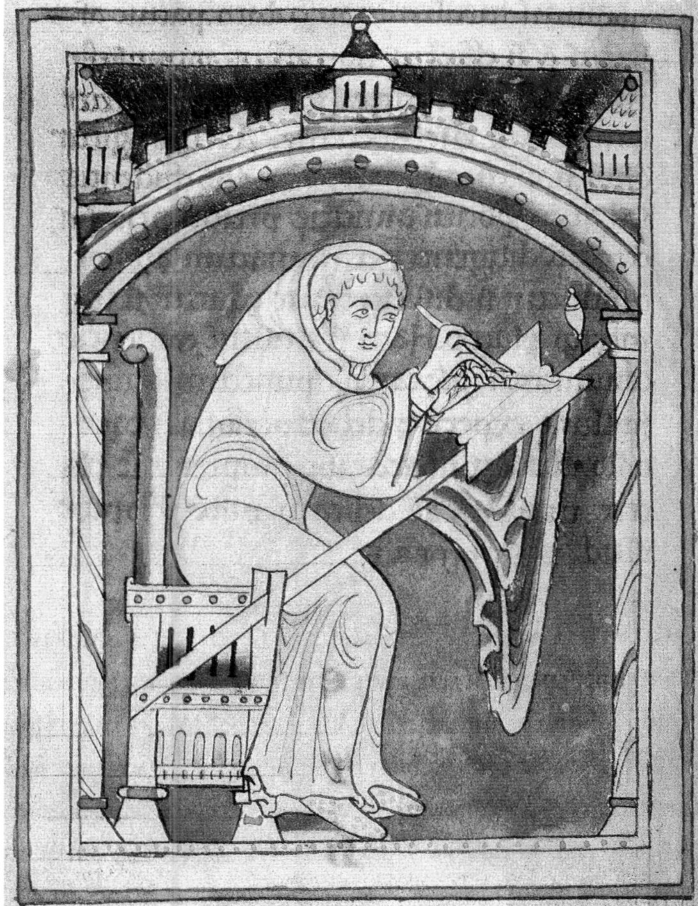

*Above* Laurence, prior of Durham 1149–54, is shown as a scribe in a contemporary manuscript of his own works, still preserved in Durham.

*1*

*2*

*3*

*4*

*5*

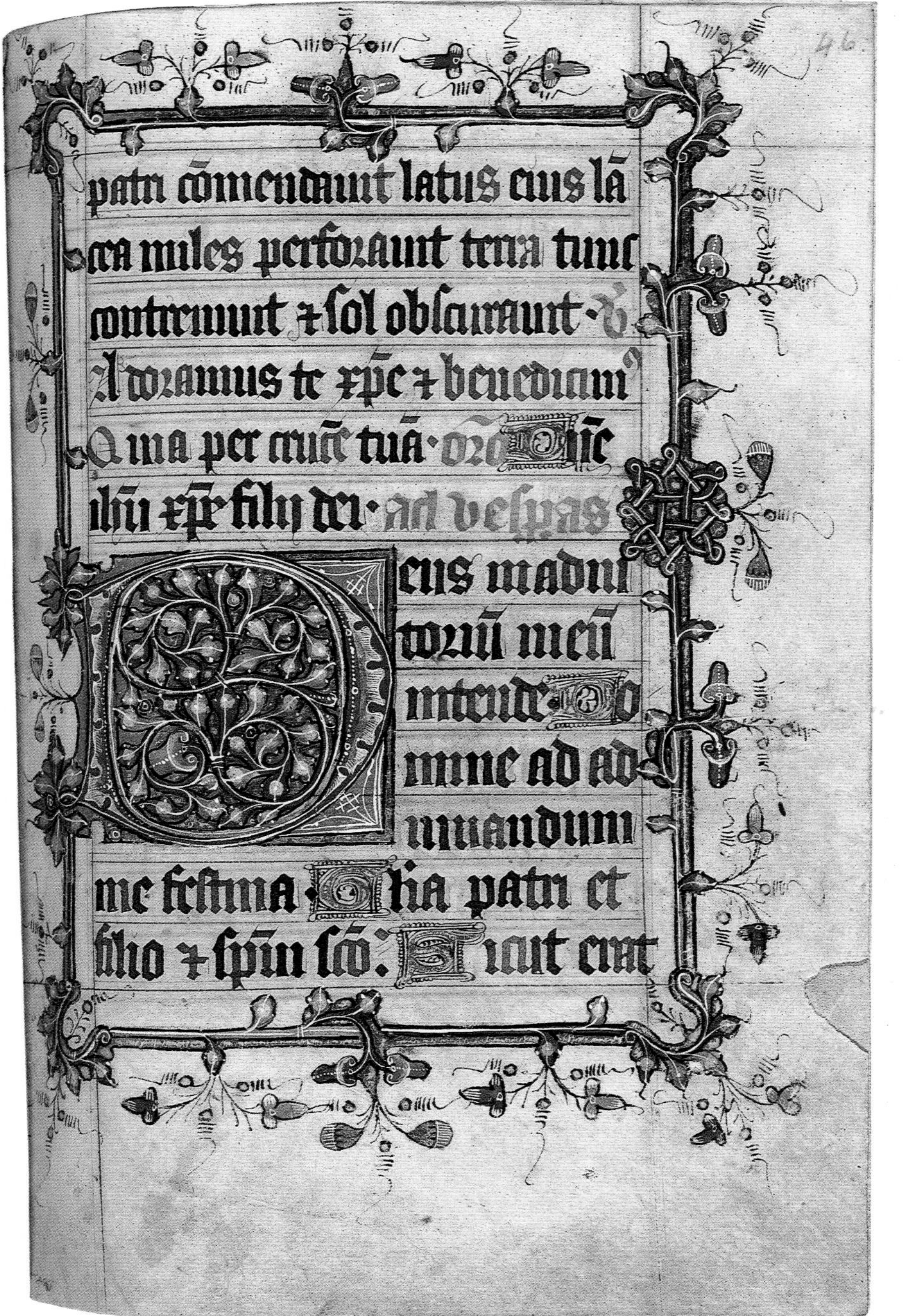

# January

6

7

8

9

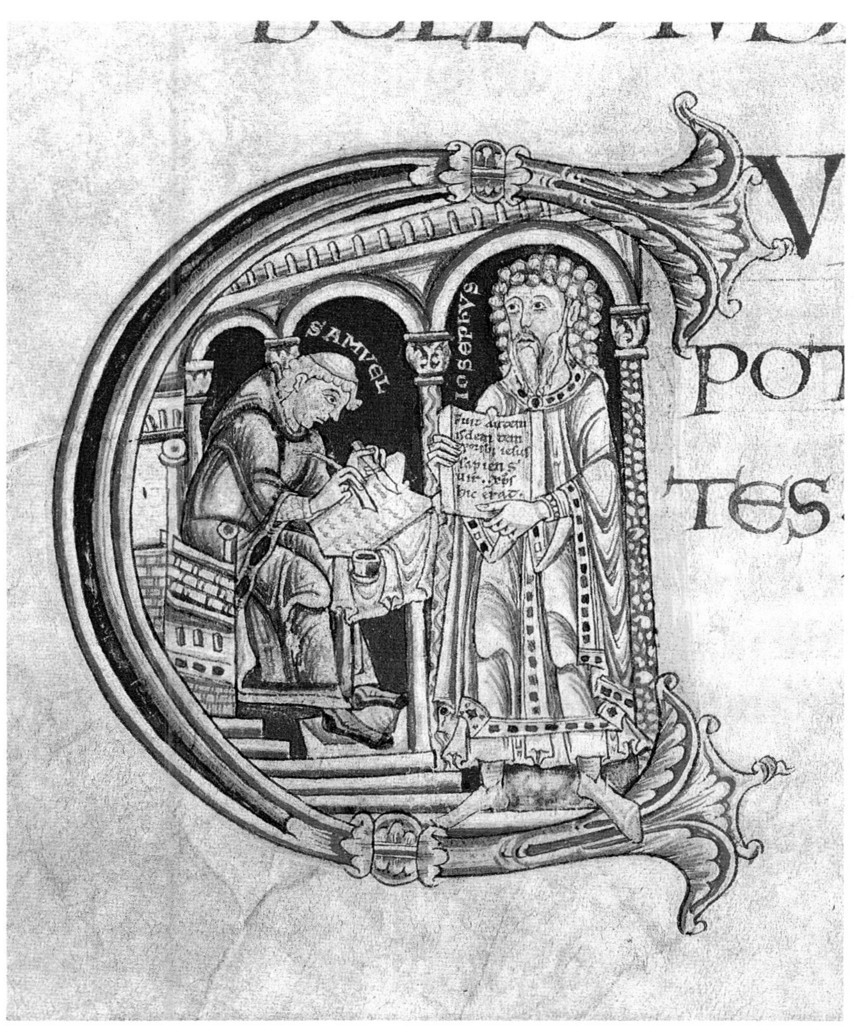


*Left* A Book of Hours illuminated in London in a professional workshop in the late fourteenth century.

*Above* A Canterbury illuminator of *c.* 1130 shows Josephus (*right*) holding a manuscript which is being copied by his scribe Samuel (*left*). Josephus wrote in the first century, but the scribe is shown as a Romanesque monk.

*10*

*11*

*12*

*13*

*14*

molestez cest leur secours joyeux Cest le repos
de tous les langoureux Cest leur salut et
remede courtoys. Et pour brief dire vng
tresaffectueux. Lit prepare au fil du roy des
roys. Maistre prenez repos solacieux En
ce saint lit jours sepmaines et moys. Ecce
en celluy qui si tresdesireux Lit prepare
au fil du roy des roys.

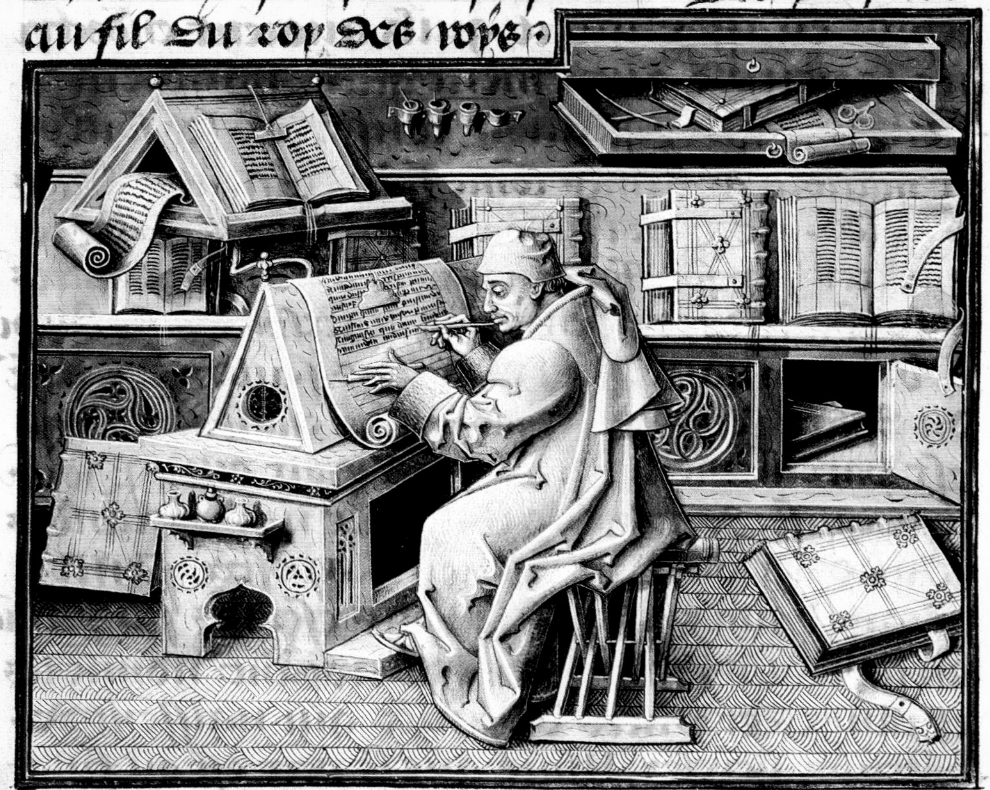

Sensieut vng petit prologue sur lassumptio de la vierge
marie translate de latin en francois. Par Jo. Milot

Valetus serviteur de ihucrist en leglise
de sarde A ses venerables freres & mes
demourans a ladene salut Je me
rammembre bien que jay souvent escript.

Jean Miélot (died 1472), a notable translator and scribe, is shown here in a study filled with a magnificent desk as well as books, manuscripts and the implements of the scribe.

# January

15

16

17

18

19

20

21

22

23

24

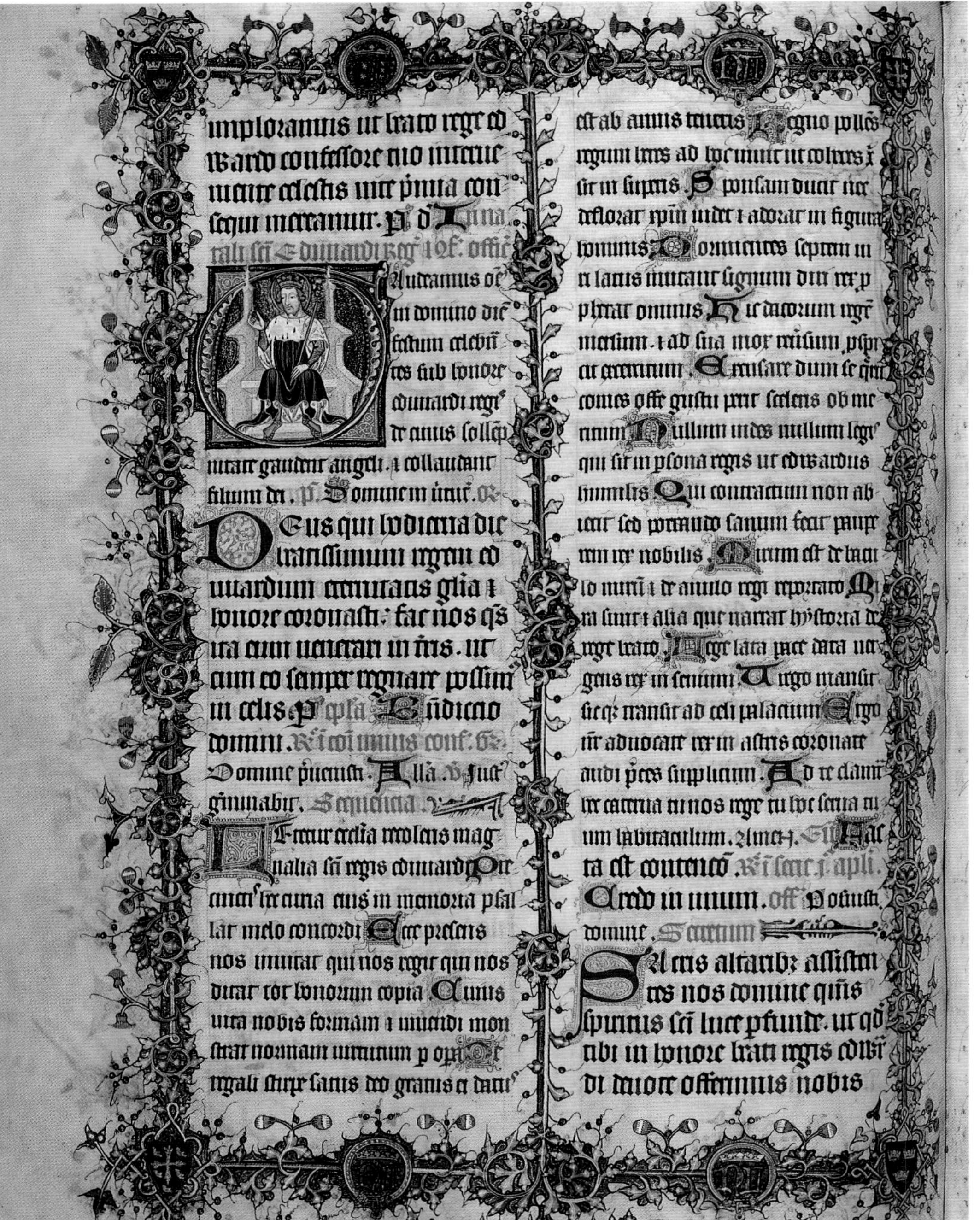

Thomas Preston spent two years as the scribe of the Litlyngton Missal made in 1383–4 for Nicholas Litlyngton, Abbot of Westminster from 1362 to 1386. The little miniature shows St Edward the Confessor, founder of Westminster Abbey.

# *January*

*25*

*26*

*27*

*28*

*29*

*30*

*31*

*All that have pleasur in this*
*booke to reade*
*Praie for my soule, and for*
*all quicke and deade*
*In the yeare of Christ* MCCCC
*seaventie and seavene*
*This worke began. Honor to*
*God in heavene.*

Colophon at the end of a fifteenth-century manuscript.

# February

MASONS

St Blaise *3 February*

St Thomas Apostle *21 December*

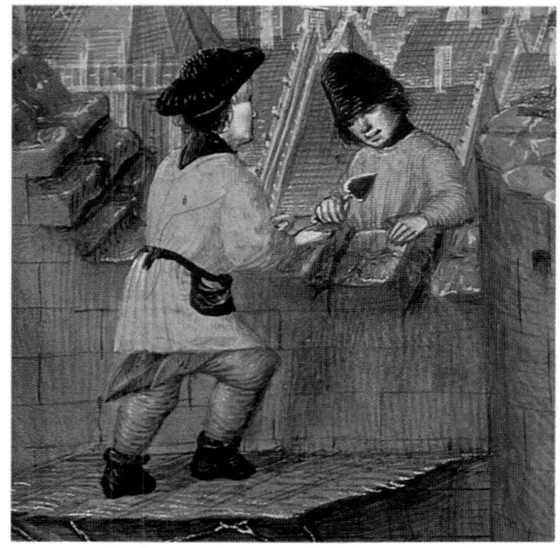

THE MEDIEVAL mason combined the skill of the modern contractor, engineer, and designer. The separation of the art of design from the knowledge of building is a post-medieval development. The design and construction of medieval buildings were rooted in the mason's craft.

His combination of skills led to greater status and power in the 13th century. The tomb of Hughes Libergier (died 1263), architect of St Nicaise at Rheims, shows him in a long robe holding his staff and surrounded by his drawing instruments. Some master masons travelled considerable distances to advise on buildings, such as the successive French and Italian masters who were invited to advise on the building of Milan Cathedral.

Some medieval architectural drawings and sketches survive. Many were made to impress the patron, but drawings were also used to choose the correct stones at the quarry for complicated tracery. Templates were widely used to cut the mouldings for piers and vaults. Profiles of mouldings were sometimes drawn out on plaster tracing floors, such as that at York Minster over the Chapter House.

Masons often visited the quarry to inspect the stone beds and to supervise the preliminary cutting of the stone. The final cutting took place in the lodge and the stones were usually put in place fully moulded. The lodge was large enough for every skilled mason to have a place to cut the more intricately moulded stones. Nearby would be the tracing house where designs were drawn and the forge where cutting tools were sharpened.

Masons in the Middle Ages built castles and great churches for the display of temporal and spiritual power. These great buildings, sometimes tall and fragile-looking, were frequently triumphs of skill over probability. Today they survive as the most memorable remains of the medieval world.

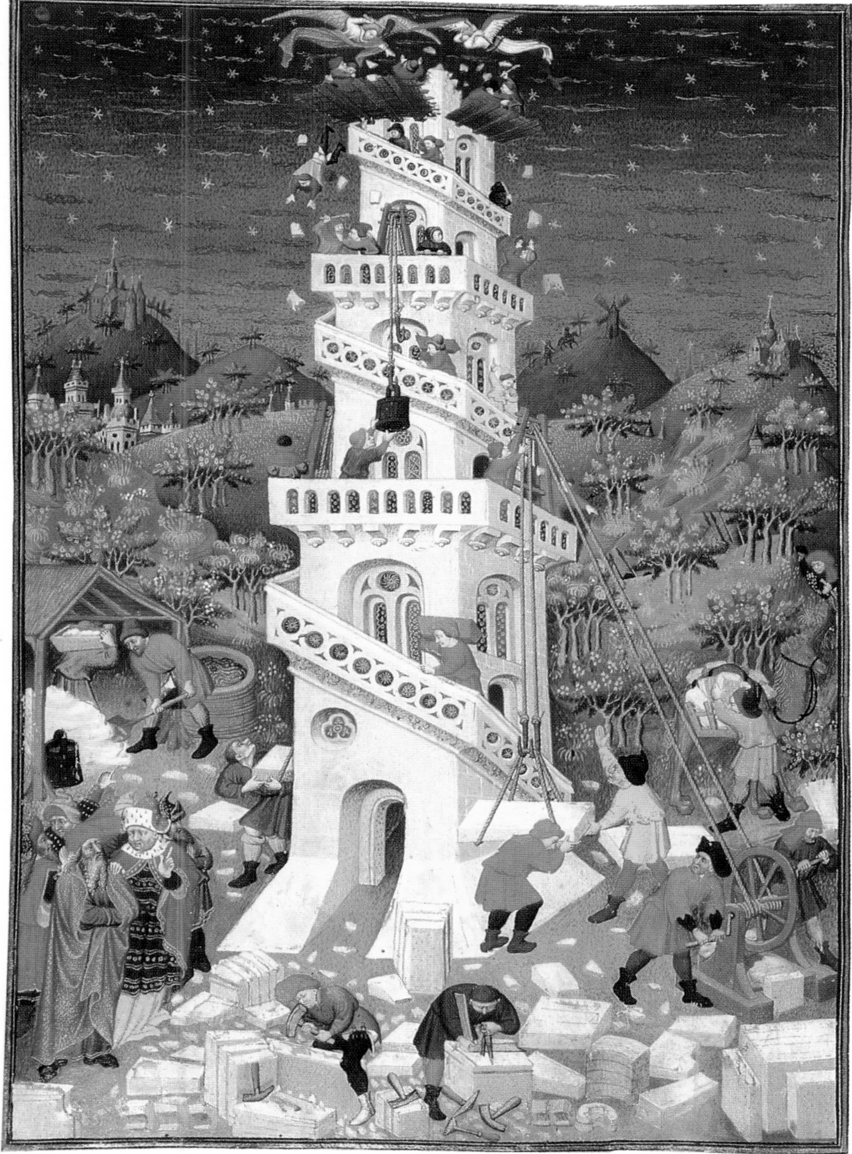

*Above left* Fifteenth-century masons at work.

*Above* The depiction of the building of the Tower of Babel in the fifteenth-century Bedford Hours.

1

2

3

4

5

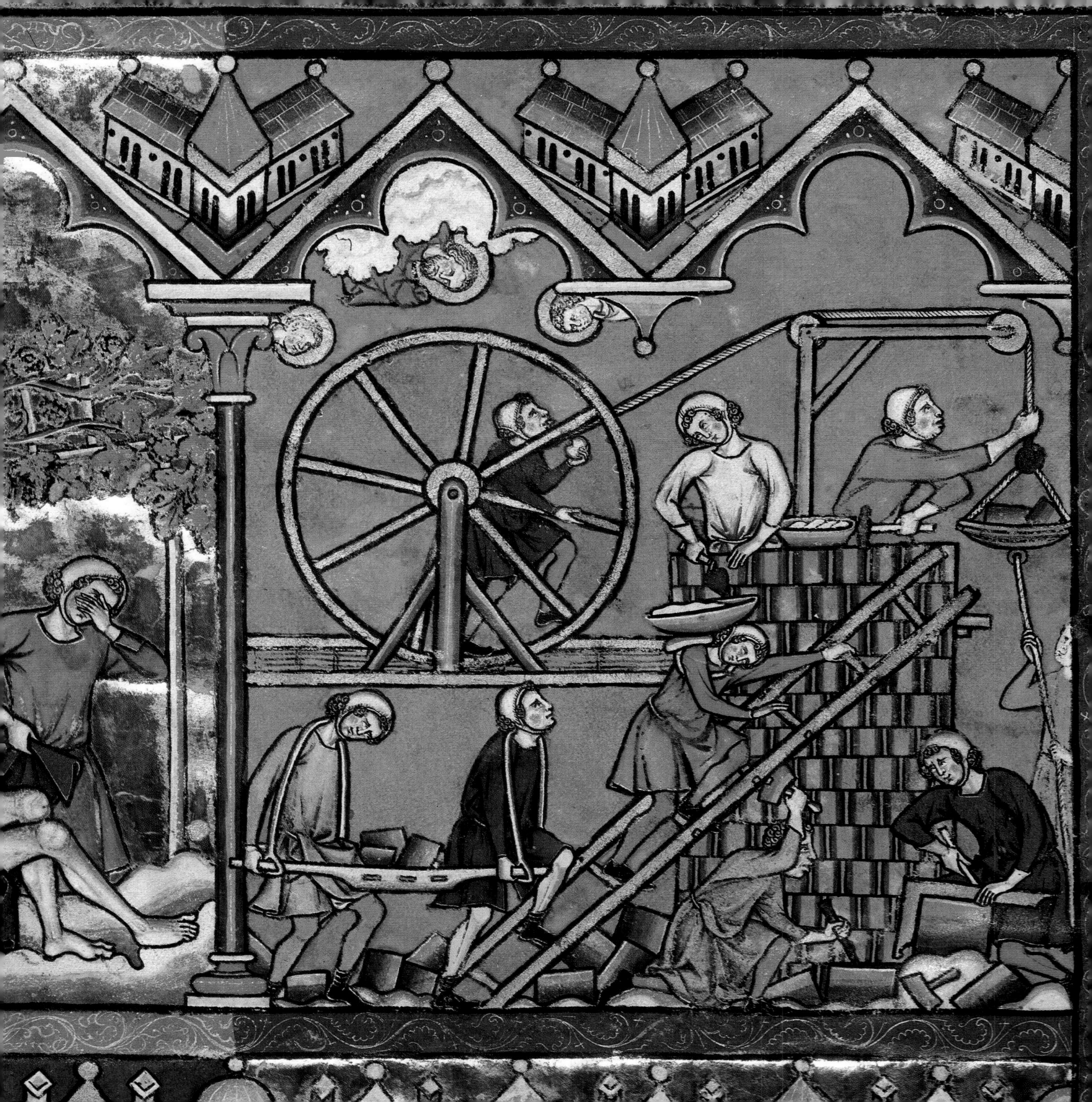

# February

*10*

*6*

*11*

*7*

*12*

*8*

*13*

*9*

*14*

The use of the wheel to raise stone and the other implements of the mason is well shown in this illumination.

# February

*15*

*16*

*17*

*18*

*19*

*20*

*21*

*22*

*23*

*24*

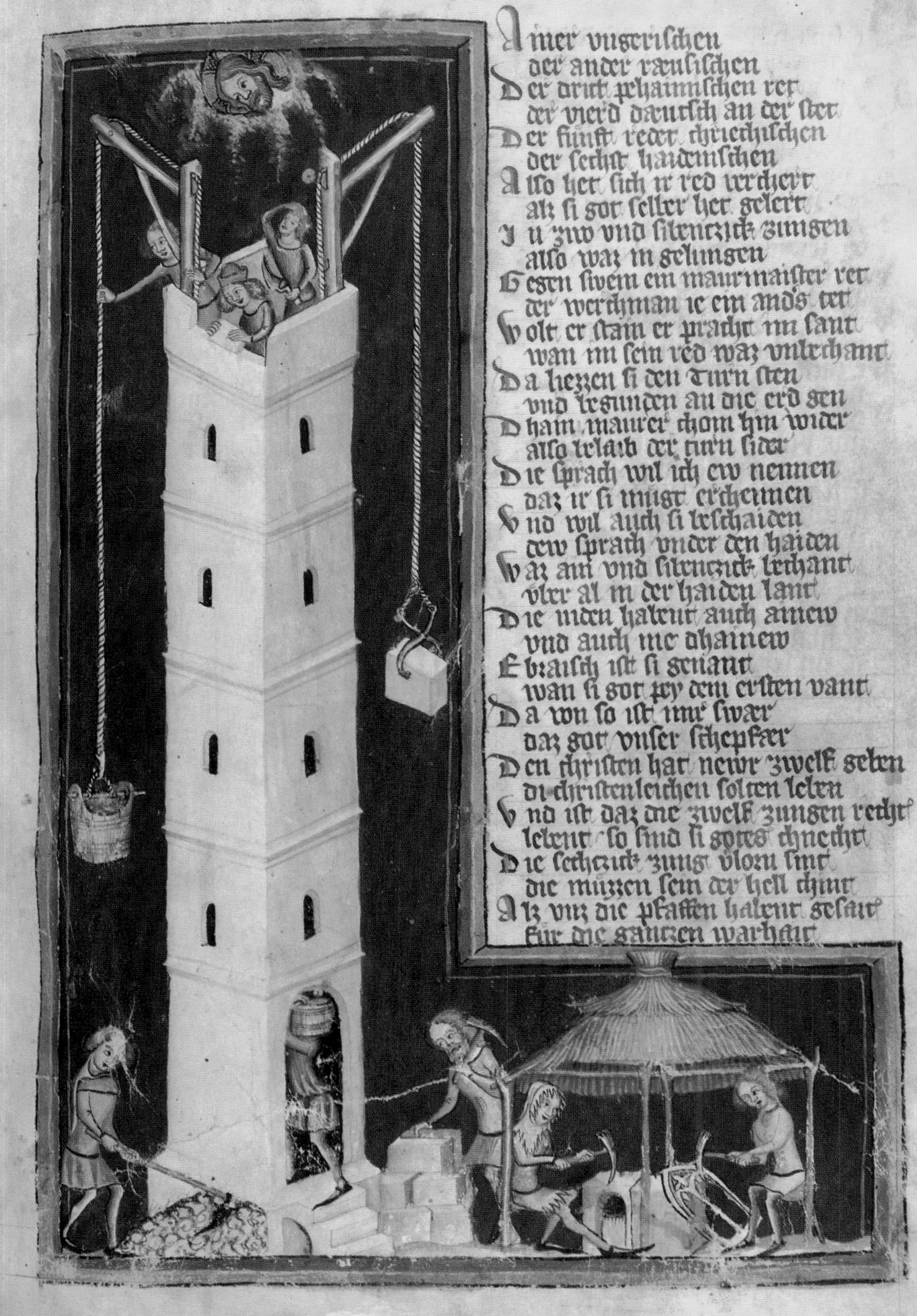

Hoists, sometimes with pincers, were used to raise materials to the top of buildings. This fourteenth-century German illumination shows a thatched wooden shelter where the sculptors carve stone and a window.

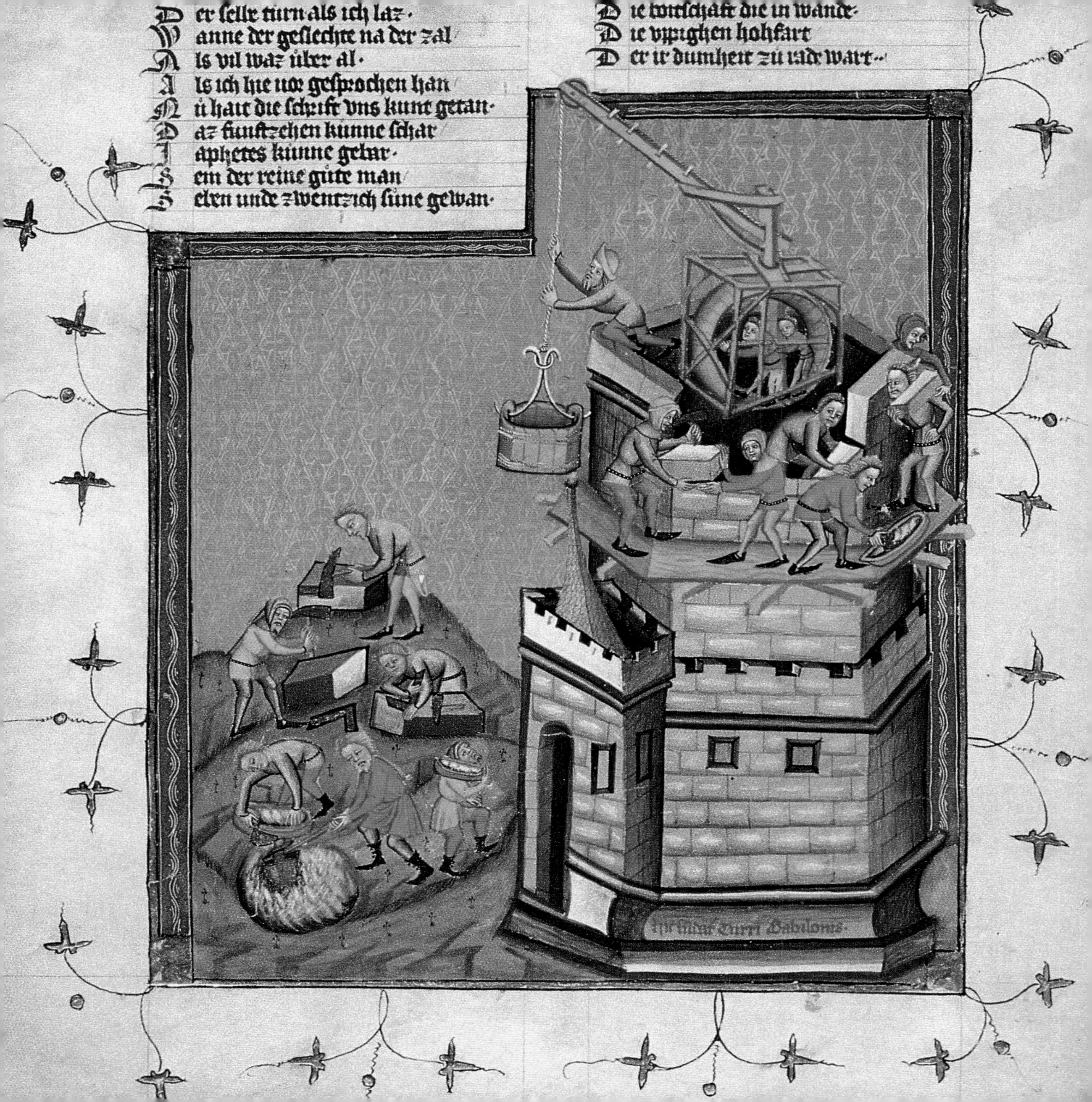

Der selbe turn als ich laz.
Wanne der geslechte na der zal
Als vil waz über al.
Als ich hie vor gesprochen han
Nů hait die schrift vns kunt getan.
Daz funftzehen kunne schar
Iaphetes kunne gebar.
Sem der reine gůte man
Selen unde zwentzich sune gewan.
Die wirtschaft die in wande.
Die vppighen hohfart
Der ir dumheit zu rade wart.

# *February*

*25*

*26*

*27*

*28*

*29*

These masons have gained access to the top of this Tower of Babel by climbing up internal stairs. At the top they have an ingenious man-operated crane.

*He addressed himself to the procuring of stone beyond the sea. He constructed ingenious machines for loading and unloading ships, and for drawing cement and stones. He delivered moulds for shaping the stones to the sculptors who were assembled, and diligently prepared other things of the same kind.*

William of Sens, master mason of the new choir of Canterbury Cathedral.

# March
## SCULPTORS

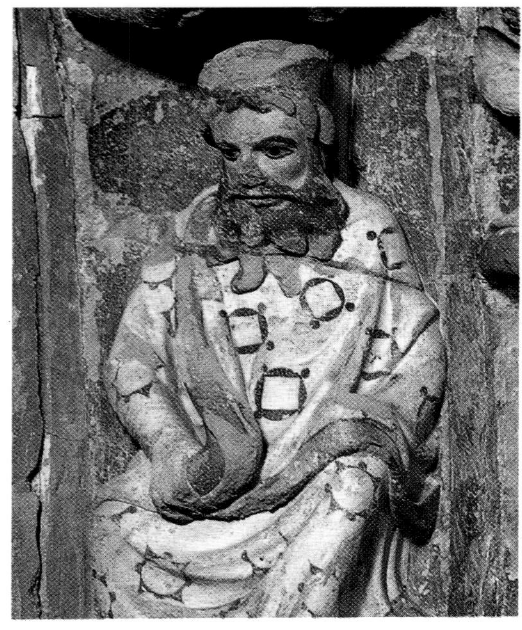

STONE CARVING was carried out both in the quarry and the mason's lodge and so it is difficult to say when the medieval sculptor became an independent specialist. By the late thirteenth century the term *magister* is used in building accounts to distinguish a separate craft. At Exeter in 1323–4 a sculptor was brought from London to carve images, even though the regular workforce of stone masons was carving decoration on the vaulting of the Cathedral.

The distinction between masons and sculptors was not always clear. In the account for the Eleanor Crosses made in 1291–4 to commemorate the resting places of the coffin of Queen Eleanor, wife of Edward I, Alexander of Abingdon, who seems to have been primarily a figure sculptor, is described indiscriminately as imaginator or cementarius. It is also known that some of the statues for the Eleanor cross at Northampton were taken there ready-carved from the sculptor's workshop rather than carved on site. However, other sculptures in churches were clearly carved in the building rather than transported from the workshop or the quarry.

The stone block was first marked with chalk and roughed out in general shape. Figure statues were often hollowed out at the back to make them lighter. The sculptor would use increasingly finer tools. He would begin with an axe or hammer and progress to chisels or drills for the finer work, ultimately tooling the surface with a fine chisel or file. It is possible that on some major schemes with complex narrative scenes there was a range of sculptors involved from the master, who planned the whole sequence, to lesser sculptors, who carved details of varying difficulty or specialisation. The tombs and effigies that survive in many English parish churches are one of the lasting memorials of the medieval sculptor's art.

*Above left* Much original colour remains on this thirteenth-century figure from the portal of Lausanne Cathedral in Switzerland.

*Right* A late thirteenth-century Spanish wooden image of the Virgin and Child which retains much of its colouring.

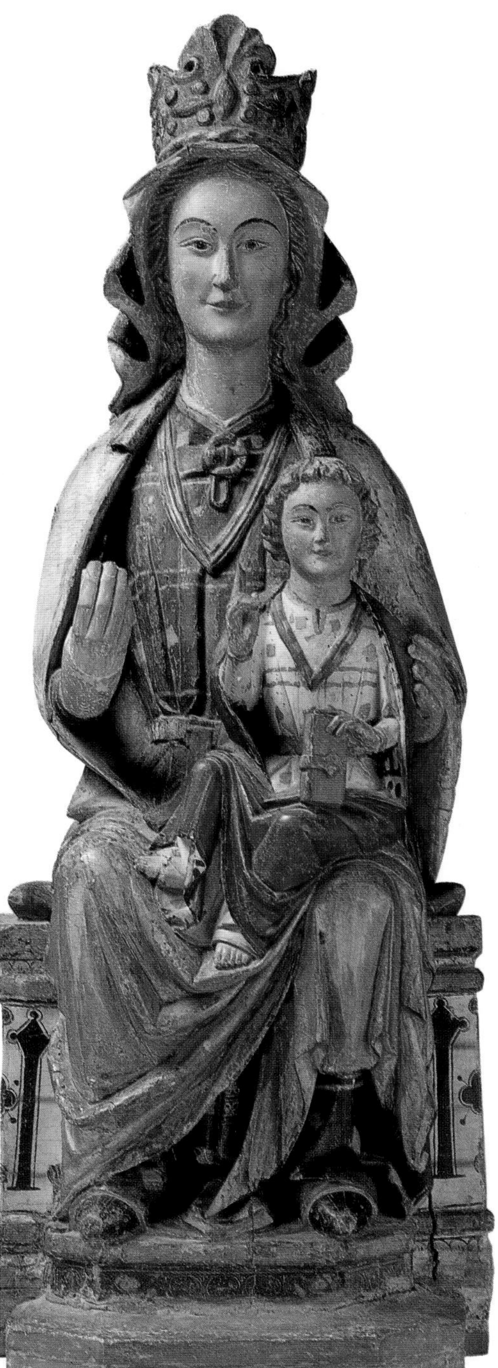

*1*

*2*

*3*

*4*

*5*

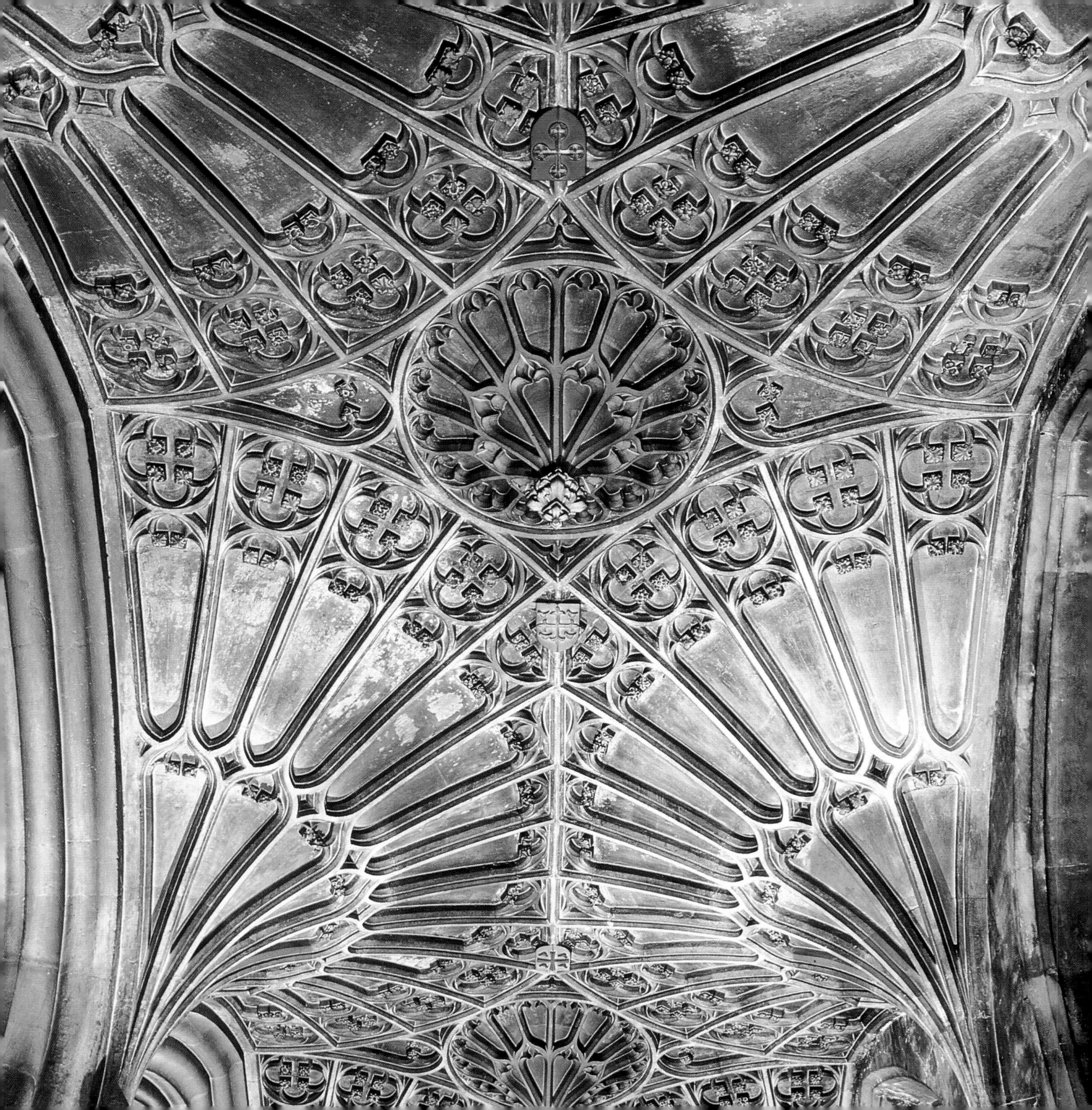

# March

6

7

8

9

Robert and William Vertue, who designed these elaborate fan vaults at Bath Abbey in the early sixteenth century, alleged that they would be better than any in England or France.

10

11

12

13

14

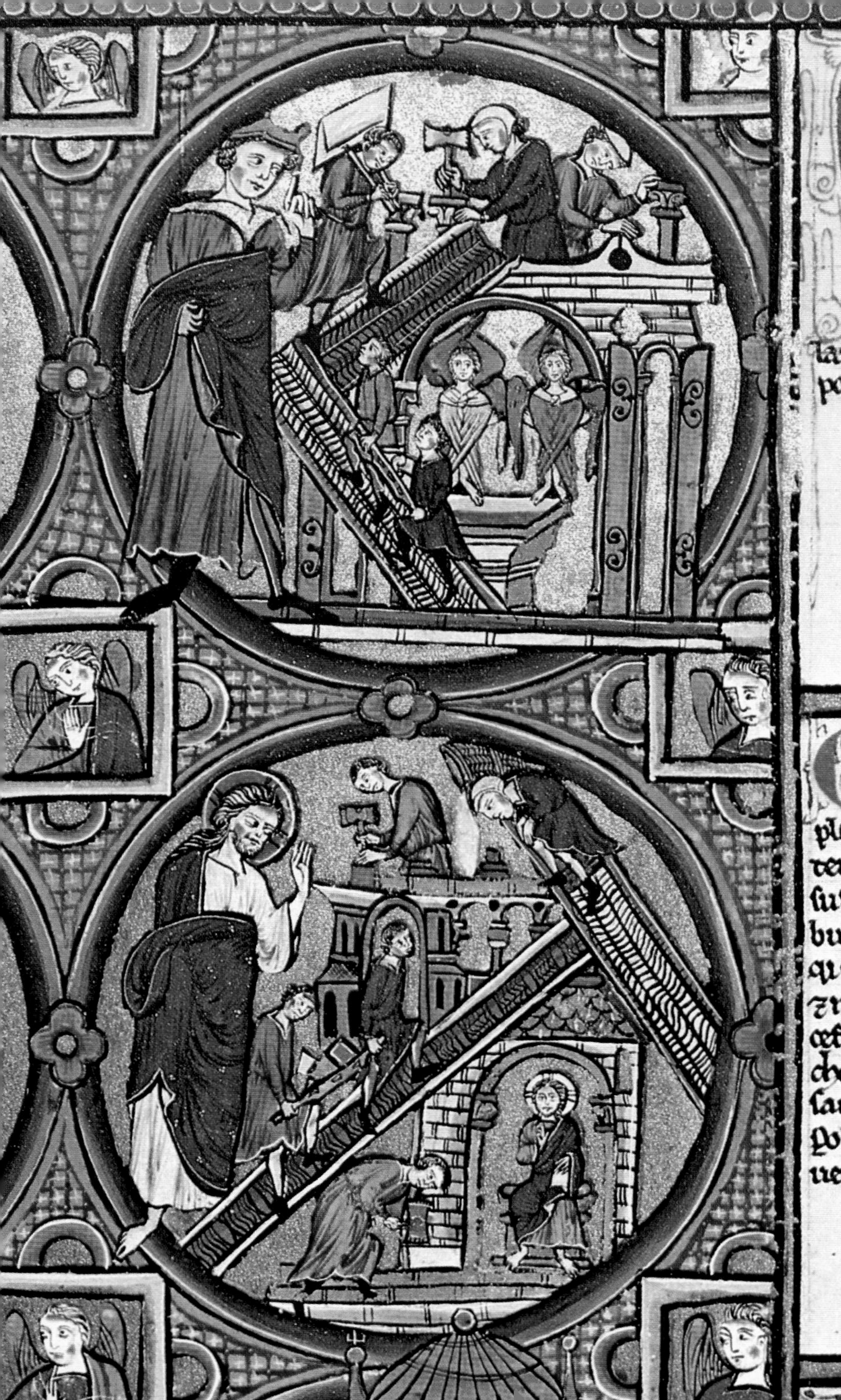

# March

15

16

17

Masons carrying material and setting capitals in the upper part of a building.

*The other image shall be a counterfeit of a lady lying in her open surcoat with two angels holding a pillow under her head and two little dogs at her feet.*

From the contract for the alabaster effigy of the wife of Ralph Greene at Lowick, Northants, in 1418–9.

18

19

20

21

22

23

24

25

26

27

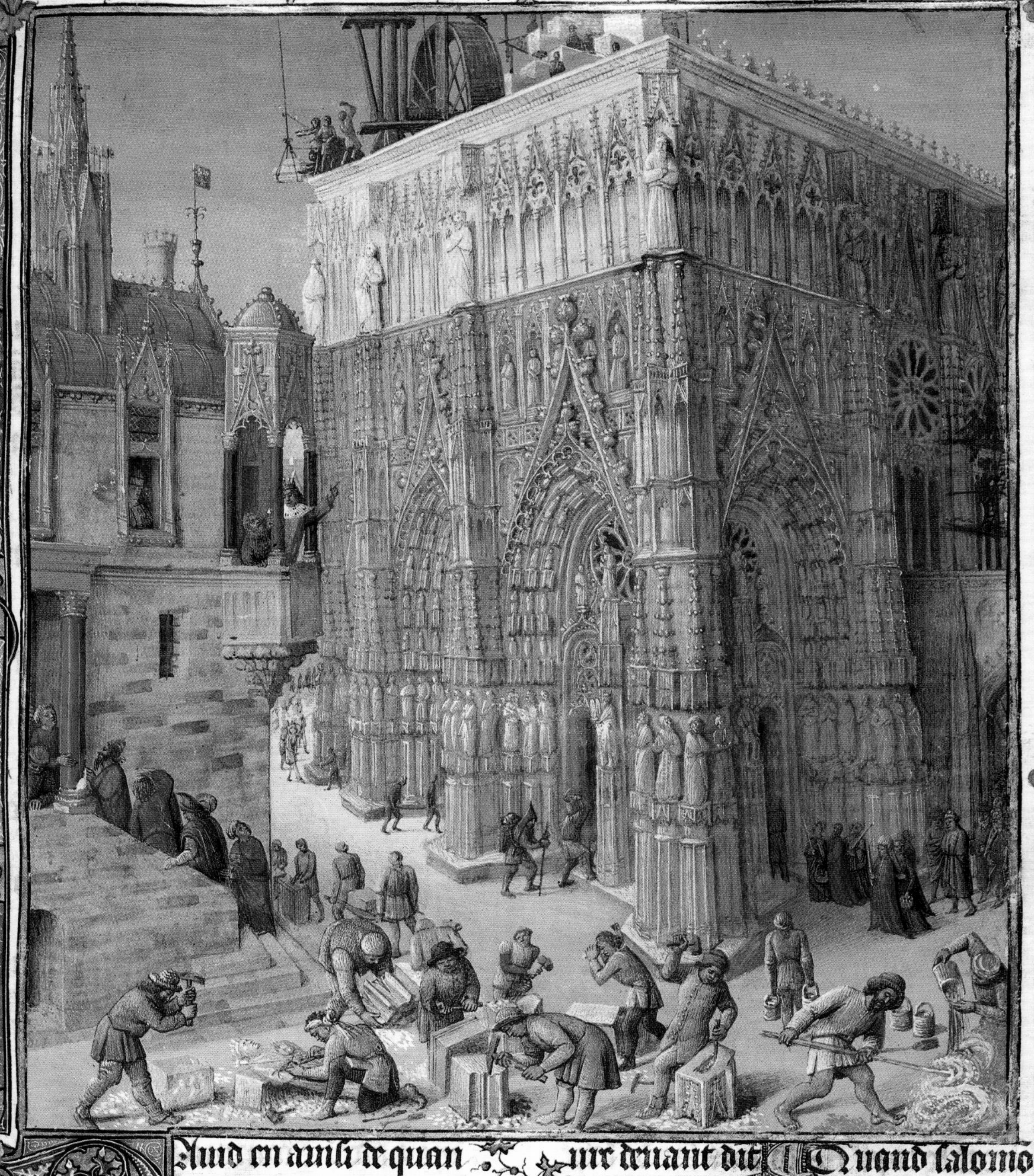

*Left* This fifteenth-century miniature by Jean Fouquet shows the Temple of Jerusalem being built. It is shown as a Gothic cathedral.

*Right* The master mason, holding his square, demonstrates to the patron of the building how hard the craftsmen are plying their tools.

# March

28

29

30

31

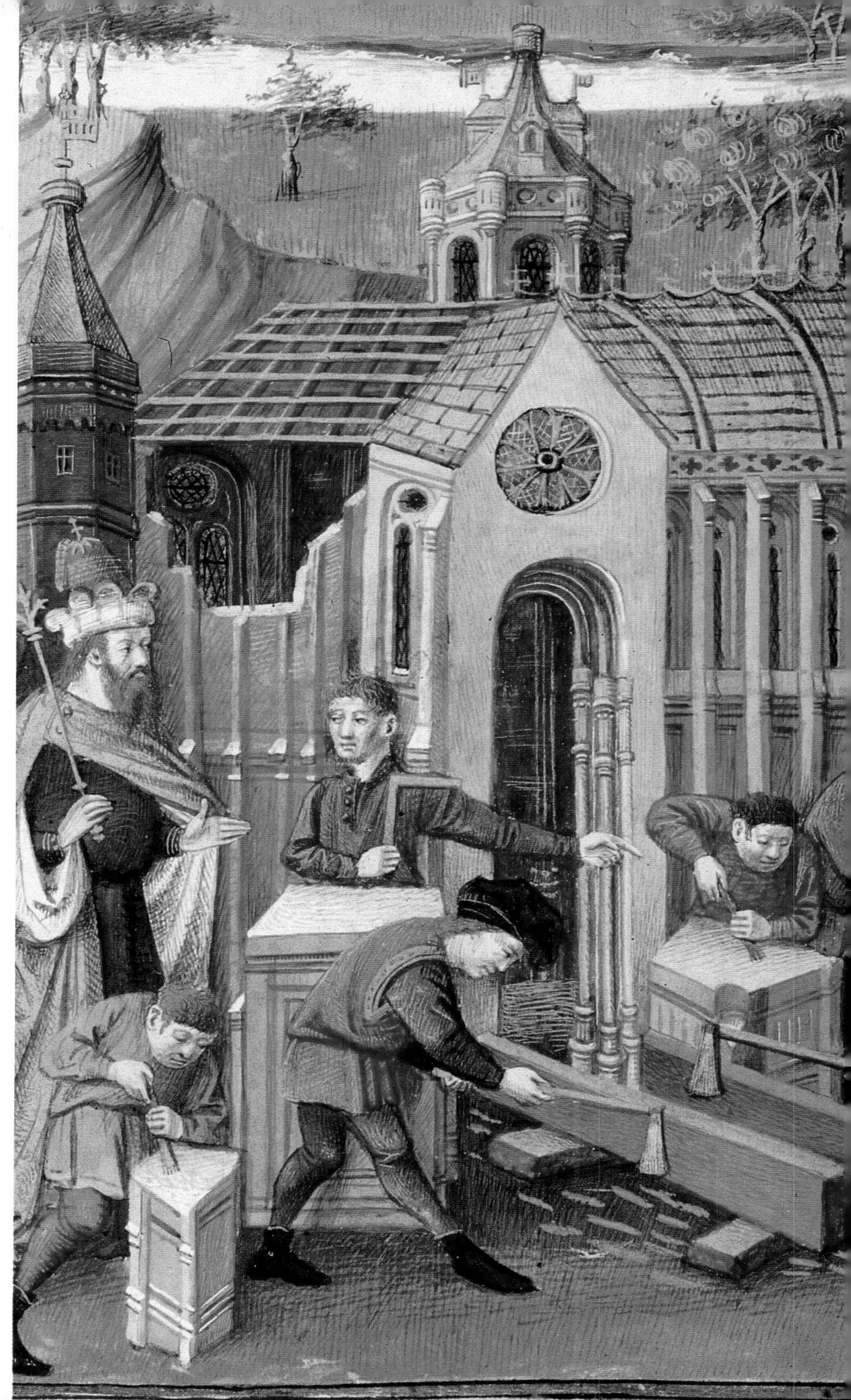

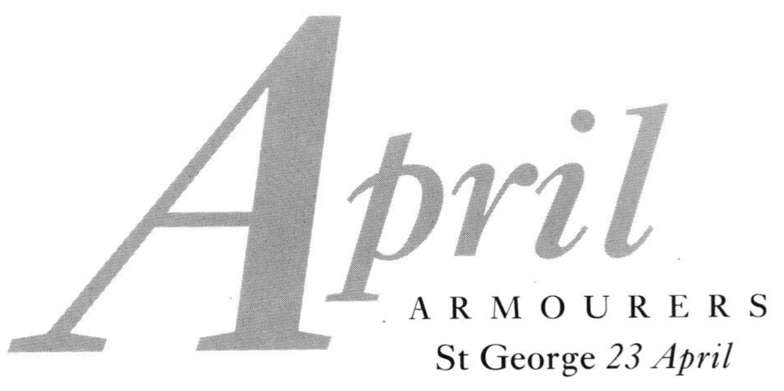


## ARMOURERS

St George *23 April*

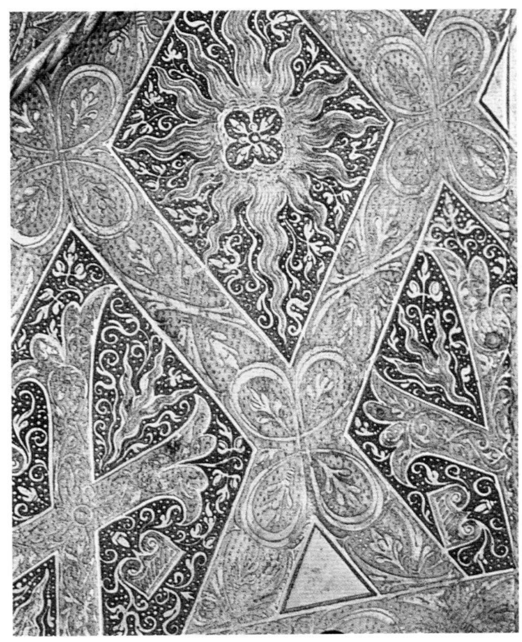

THE WORK of the medieval armourer was very often a matter of life and death for the medieval knight. Armour made of circular links of mail, which can be seen in the illumination by Matthew Paris, was flexible and relatively comfortable to wear. It was the main form of armour in the early Middle Ages but very little is known about the craftsmen who made it. The effectiveness of the longbow and crossbow led to the development of plate armour, whose greatest period lasted from the fourteenth to the seventeenth century.

The craft of armour-making needed patronage, resources such as charcoal and iron, and also swift-flowing water to drive the wheels that produced the power for the heavy hammers. Italy and Germany were the two main centres of armour manufacture. That made in Milan was widely exported and, within Italy, Milan was only rivalled as a centre by Brescia. In Germany the production of armour was concentrated in the Rhine-Westphalia region and in southern Germany, in the cities of Augsburg and Nuremberg.

The decoration of armour, particularly that commissioned by Emperors and Princes, was of the highest artistic quality. The techniques used include engraving, gilding, etching and painting. One of the techniques that gave some German armours of the late fifteenth century a look of great luxury was *goldschmelz*. Shallow patterns were etched on the blued surface and this surface was then gilded to give a sumptuous gold and blue effect.

The sixteenth century albums which record the armours made by particular armourers provide valuable information. The sketch book of Jorg Sörg, made between 1548 and 1563, tells us not only the names of the Augsburg armourers but also identifies their patrons among the noble families of Germany, Spain and Italy.

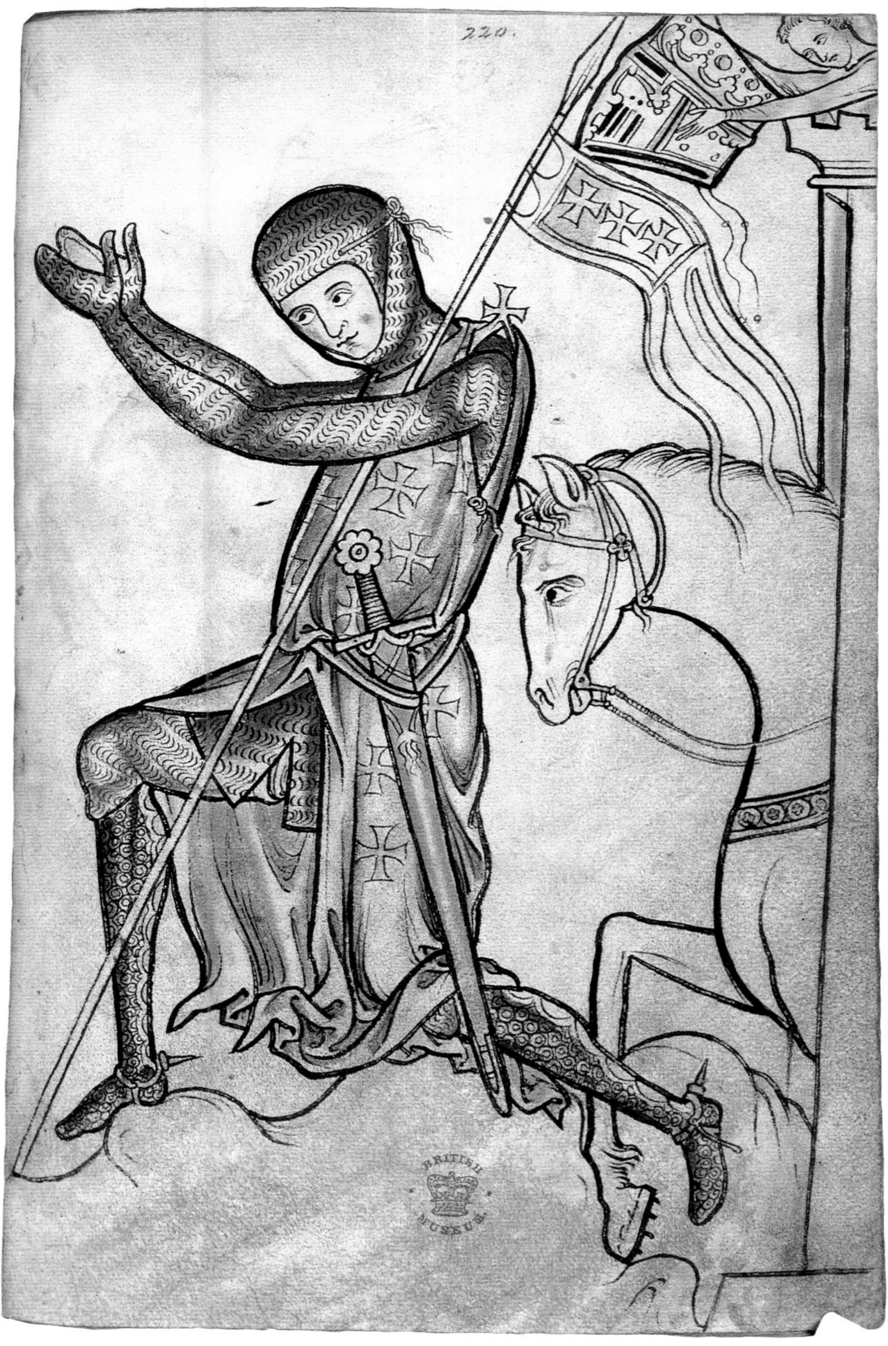

1

2

3

4

*Above left* A detail of the armour made for the future Philip II of Spain, 1551.

*Left* The mail armour and surcoat of a thirteenth-century knight, shown by Matthew Paris of St Albans *c.* 1250.

# April

*5*

*6*

*7*

*8*

*9*

*10*

*11*

*12*

*13*

*14*

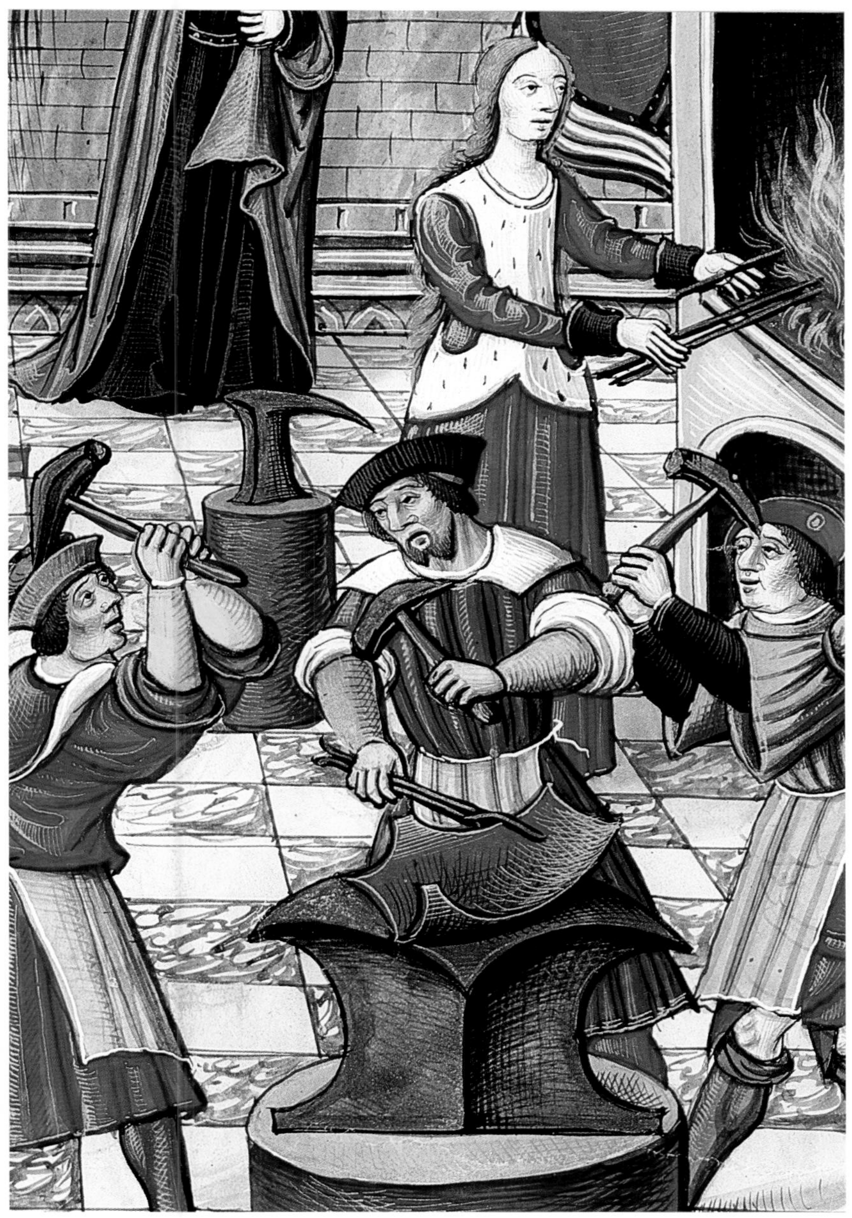

Armourers beating out a breast plate on an anvil. Sixteenth century.

*15*

*16*

*17*

*18*

*19*

# April

20

21

22

23

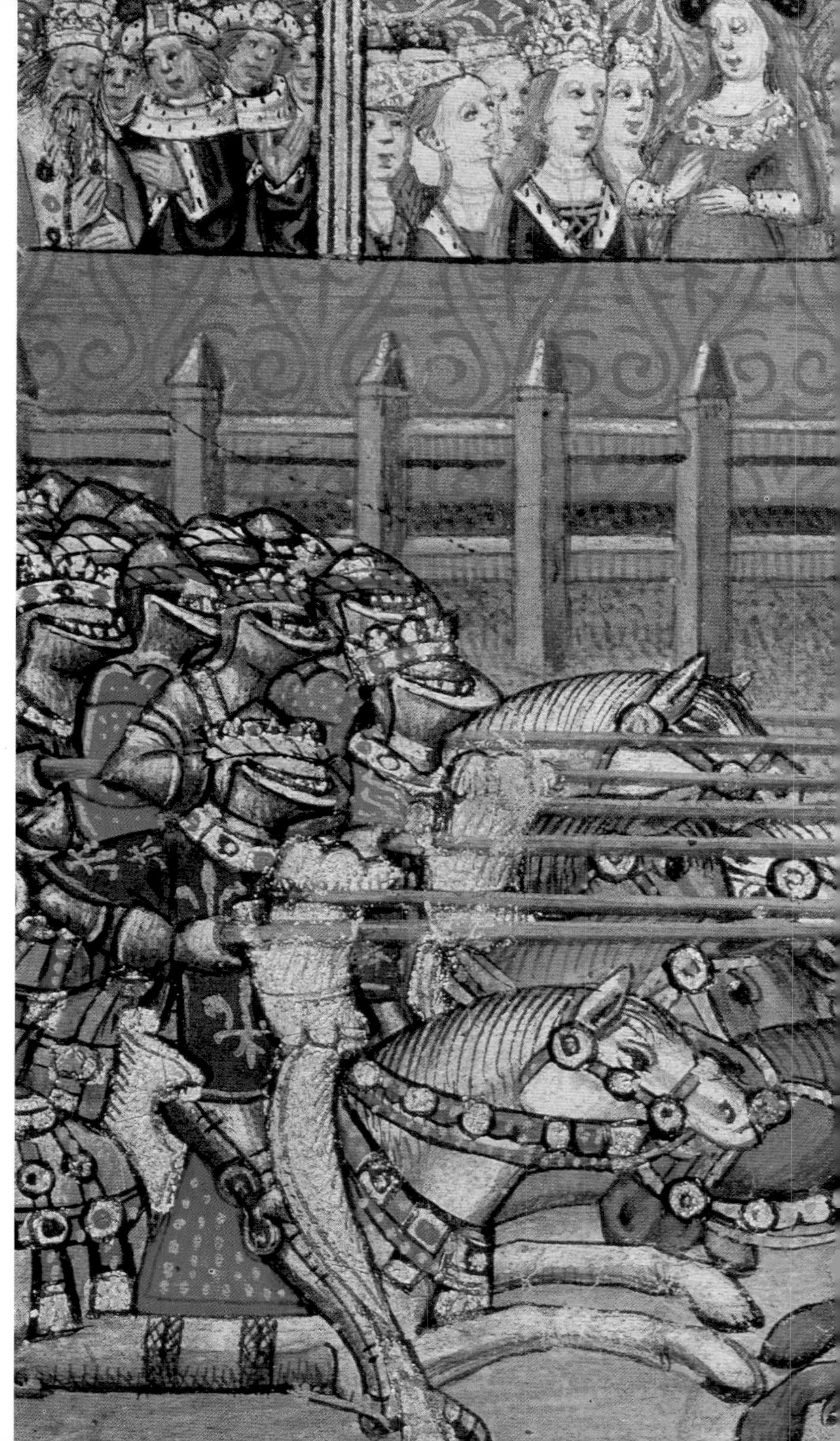

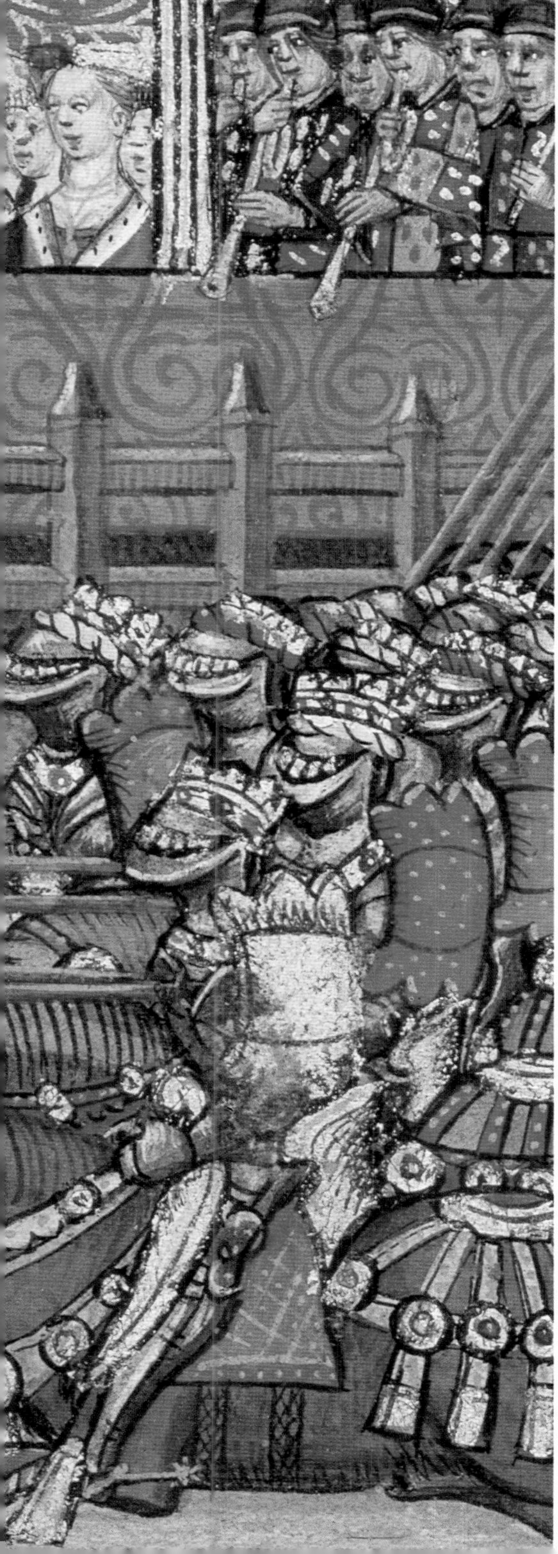

*First he laces on his* chauces *of white steel. Afterwards he dons a hauberk so valuable one could not cut a single link. When they had armed him with the hauberk, a boy laced upon his head a helmet reinforced with a gold band more shiny than a mirror.*
The arming of a knight in the *Romance of Erec.*

A joust between two companies of knights. The nobles, ladies, and minstrels watch from the safety of the stands.

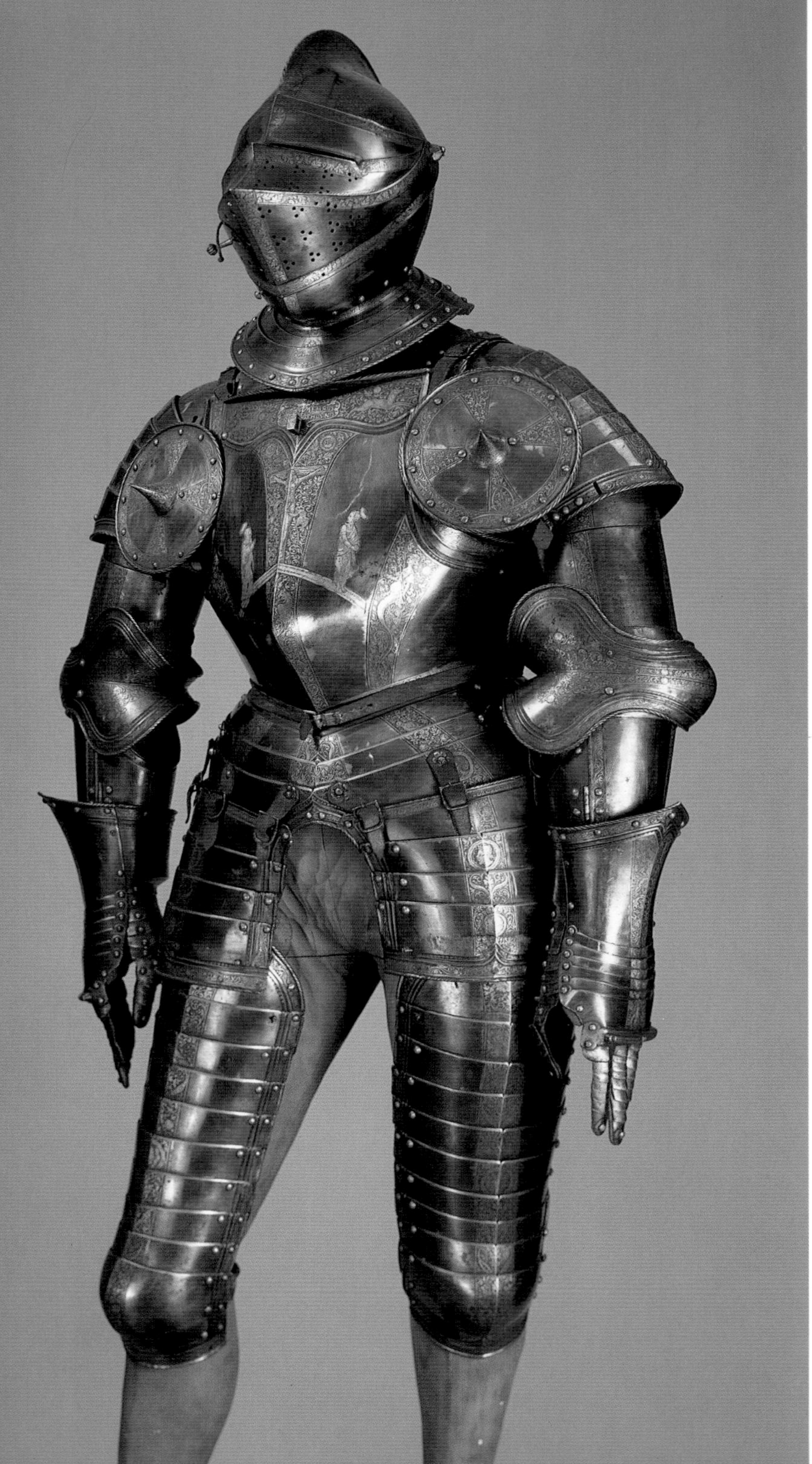

# April

24

25

26

This north German decorated half armour belonged to Johann von Rantzau (1492–1565).

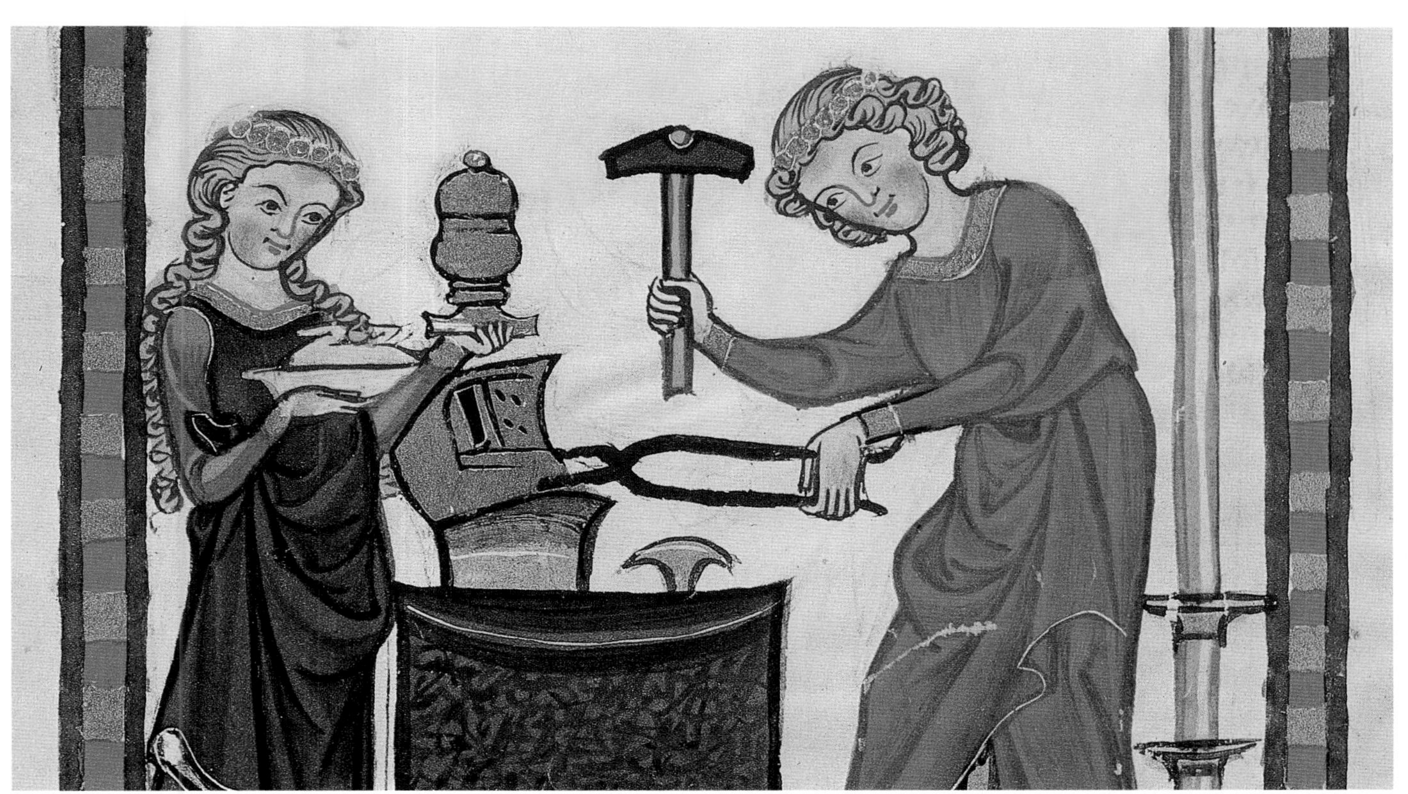

A fictional scene showing the early fourteenth-century German minstrel Hartman von Starkenberg forging a helmet.

27

29

28

30

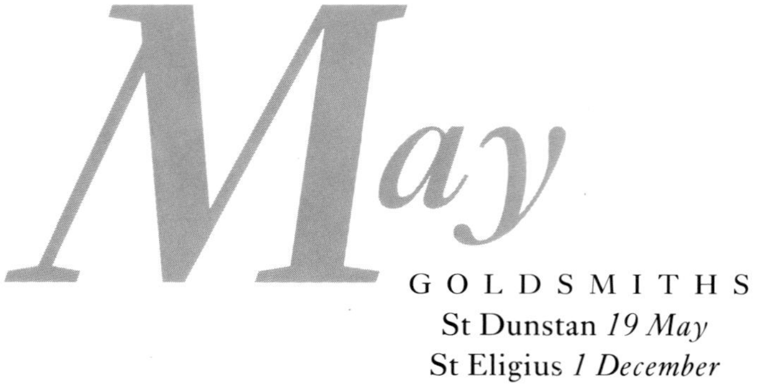


GOLDSMITHS

St Dunstan *19 May*

St Eligius *1 December*

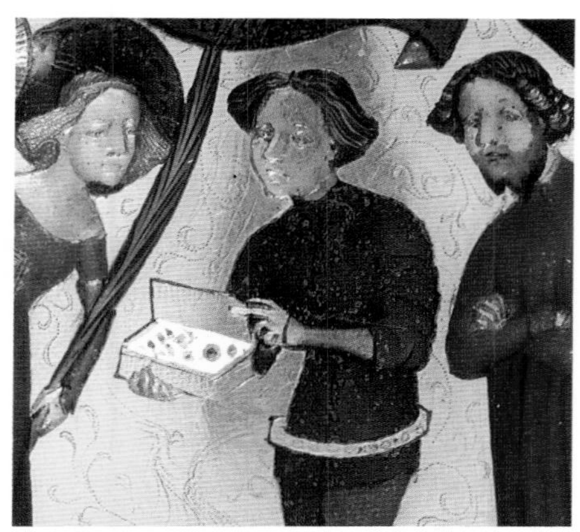

OF ALL the craftsmen the goldsmith worked upon the most precious metals, enriching them further with rare stones and engraved gems. Goldsmiths were both monastic and secular and ranged in wealth from the poor apprentices to some of the richest craftsmen of the Middle Ages. One of the finest pieces of English goldsmiths' work was the golden shrine of St Thomas à Becket at Canterbury on which, according to the Venetian ambassador in 1500, the 'gold was scarcely visible from the variety of precious stones with which it was studded, such as emeralds, diamonds, rubies and sapphires. These beauties of nature were enhanced by human skill for the gold is carved and engraved in beautiful designs both large and small.'

The patron saint of the English goldsmiths was St Dunstan (died 988). He was a Benedictine monk who was responsible for monastic reform in the tenth century. Legend relates that he tweaked the nose of the devil with his goldsmith's tongs – a story that inspired the embroidered scene of St Dunstan on the Stonyhurst chasuble (see page 13). The symbol of the goldsmith's craft was usually a brooch or covered cup. Their main products were rings, silver bowls and cups, fittings for knives and forks, spoons and occasionally seals, as well as grander objects such as crowns and chalices.

Some goldsmiths, through their wealth and their close association with coinage, were able to play a role in local administration and politics, occasionally at a national level. Sir Edmund Shaa was a prominent London goldsmith who was Engraver to the Mint, Prime Warden of the Goldsmiths' Company, and, in 1483, both made Lord Mayor and knighted for his support of Richard III. Others were less fortunate. Master Gusmin of Cologne worked for Louis, Duke of Anjou, who was a great collector of goldsmiths' work. When debts forced the Duke to melt down his treasures, Gusmin was broken-hearted and decided to sell all his goods and devote himself to God. He died in a hermitage in the mountains. Clearly some goldsmiths were distressed at the loss of their creations and not all ended their lives as successful and prosperous burghers.

*Above left* A Parisian goldsmith just before 1380 created the Royal Gold Cup whose deep blue and red translucent enamels on gold make it one of the richest pieces of medieval goldsmiths' work. This detail shows Procopius offering St Agnes jewels from a box. She refused his advances declaring she was married to Christ.

*Right* The wreath of enamelled flowers surrounded by flowers and foliage on this silver gilt spoon were produced by a Flemish goldsmith in the early fifteenth century.

*1*

*2*

*3*

*4*

*5*

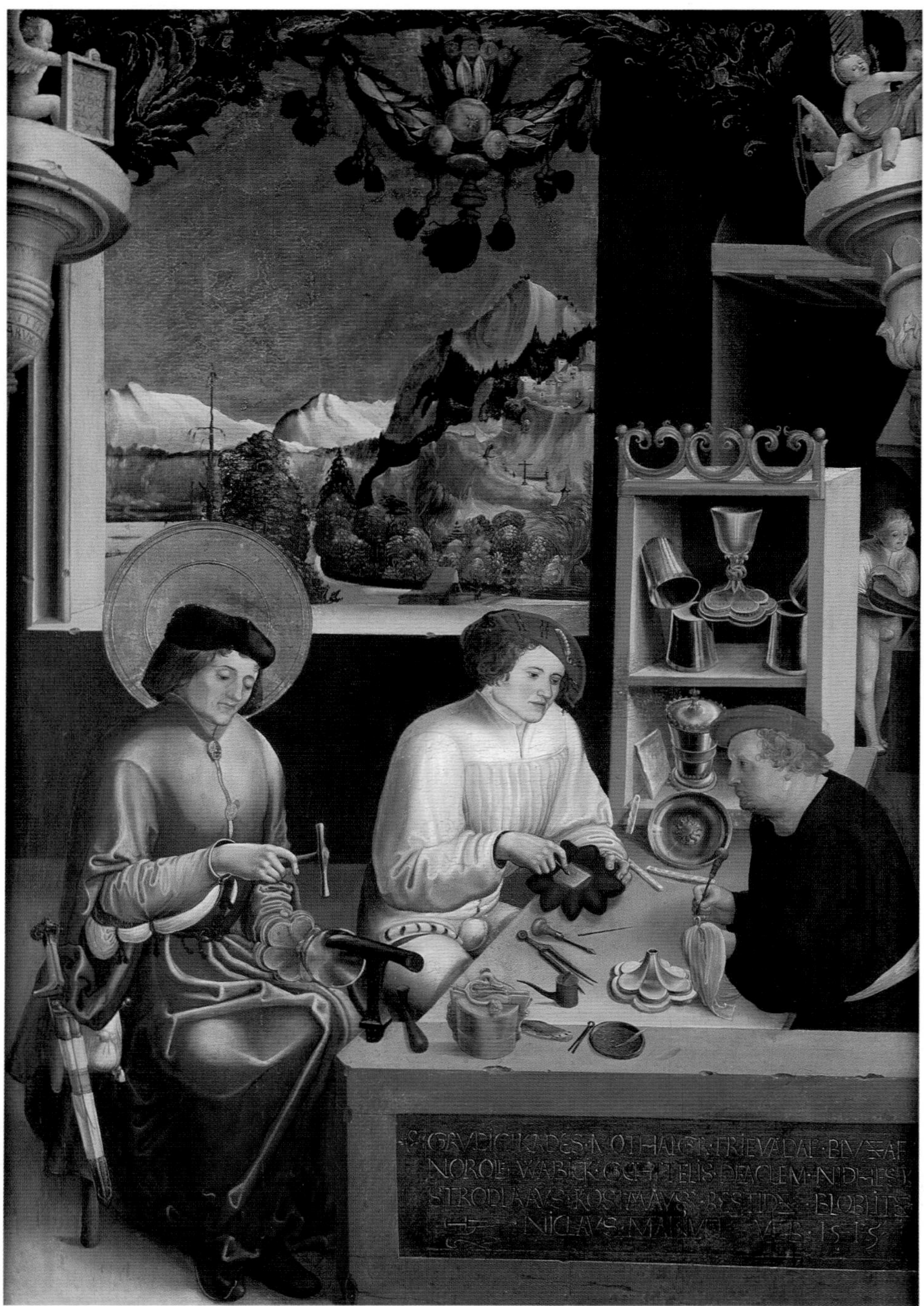

Painting of St Eligius at his work by Niclaus Manuel, 1515. This painting was ordered by the Guild of Painters and Goldsmiths of Berne, Switzerland, for the Predigerkirche. A goldsmith is shown working a ring with a chisel while the two visitors, St Eligius (with the gold halo) and his friend are hammering a silver chalice on an anvil and working the bottom of a cup.

# May

*6*

*7*

*8*

*9*

*10*

*11*

*12*

*13*

*14*

*15*

# May

16

17

18

19

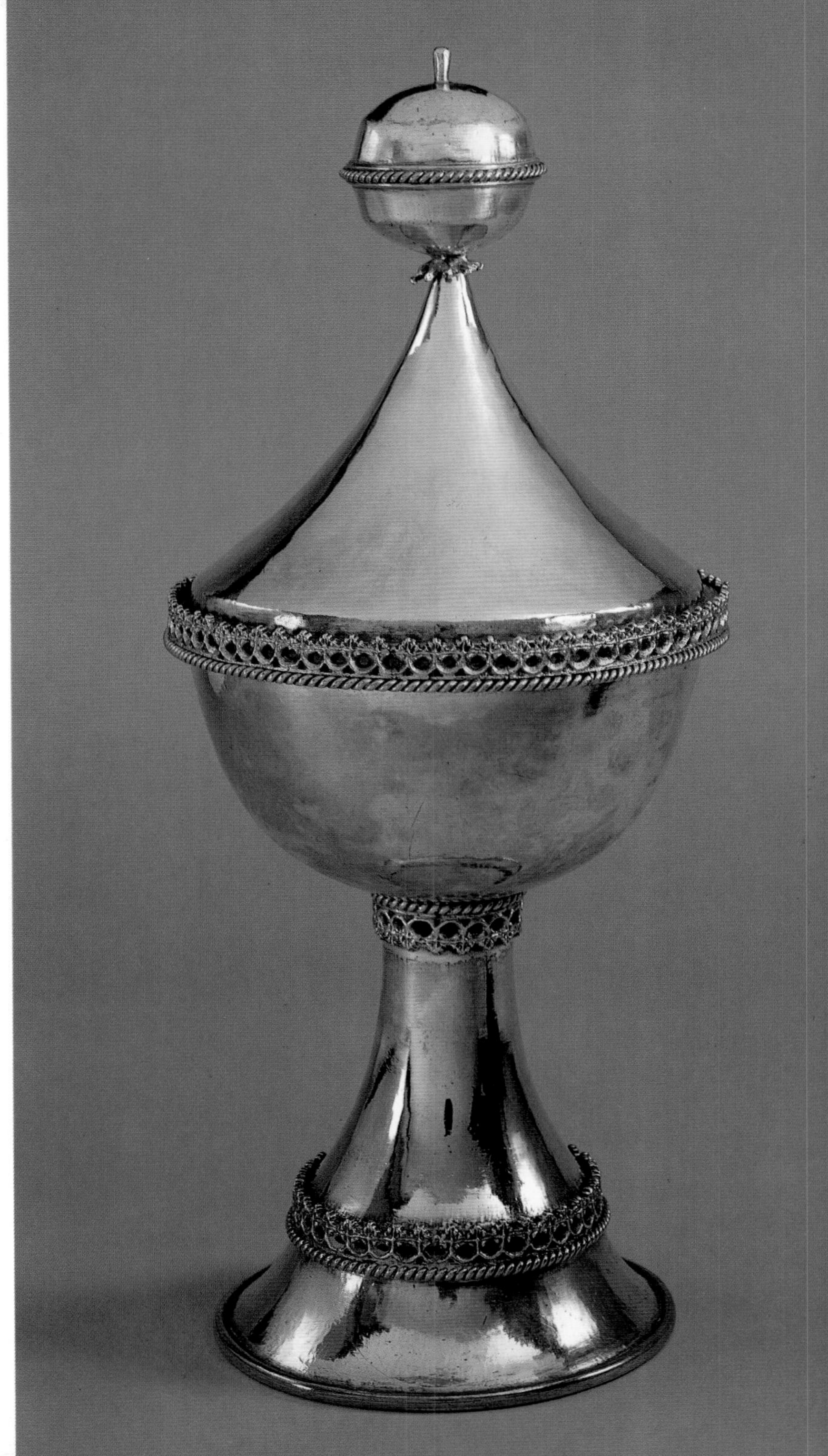

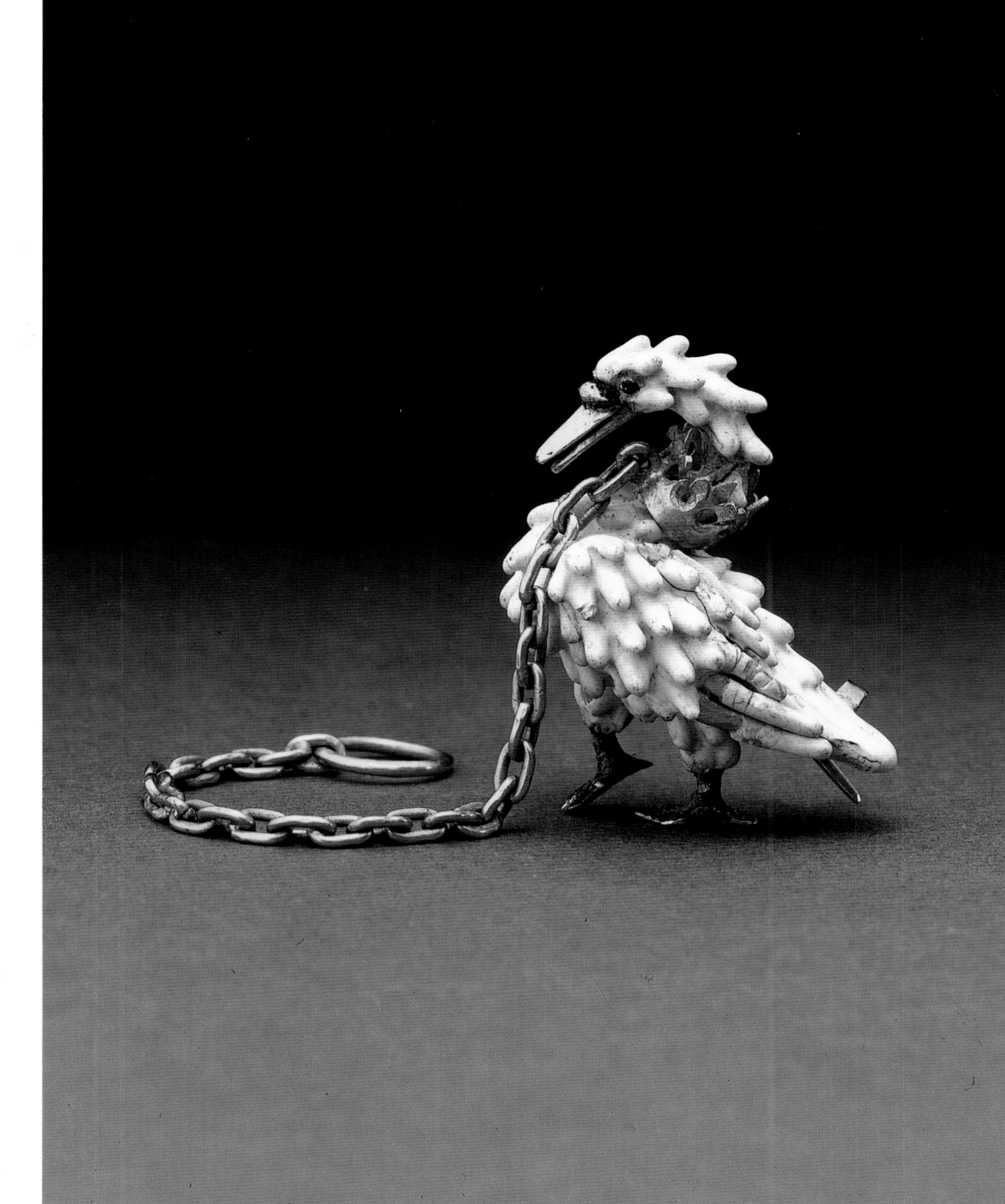

*Left* The Lacock Cup. The simple design of this silver secular cup of the first half of the fifteenth century is complemented by the bands of ornament that decorate foot, stem and lid.

*Right* The Dunstable Swan Jewel, an example of opaque white enamel over gold, probably made by a London goldsmith, *c.* 1400.

# May

*If you will diligently examine it, you will find in it whatever kinds and blends of various colours that Greece possesses: whatever Russia knows of workmanship in enamels or variety of niello: whatever Arabia adorns with repoussé or cast work, or engravings in relief: whatever gold embellishments Italy applies to various vessels or to the carving of gems and ivories: whatever France esteems in her precious variety of windows: whatever skilled Germany praises in subtle work in gold, silver, copper, iron, wood and stone.*

Theophilus on his little book *De Diversis Artibus*, 'The Various Arts'.

20

21

22

23

24

25

26

27

28

29

Silver-gilt drinking cup with a curved handle. French or German, fifteenth century. Gold, silver and silver gilt were the most prized materials for use on the table.

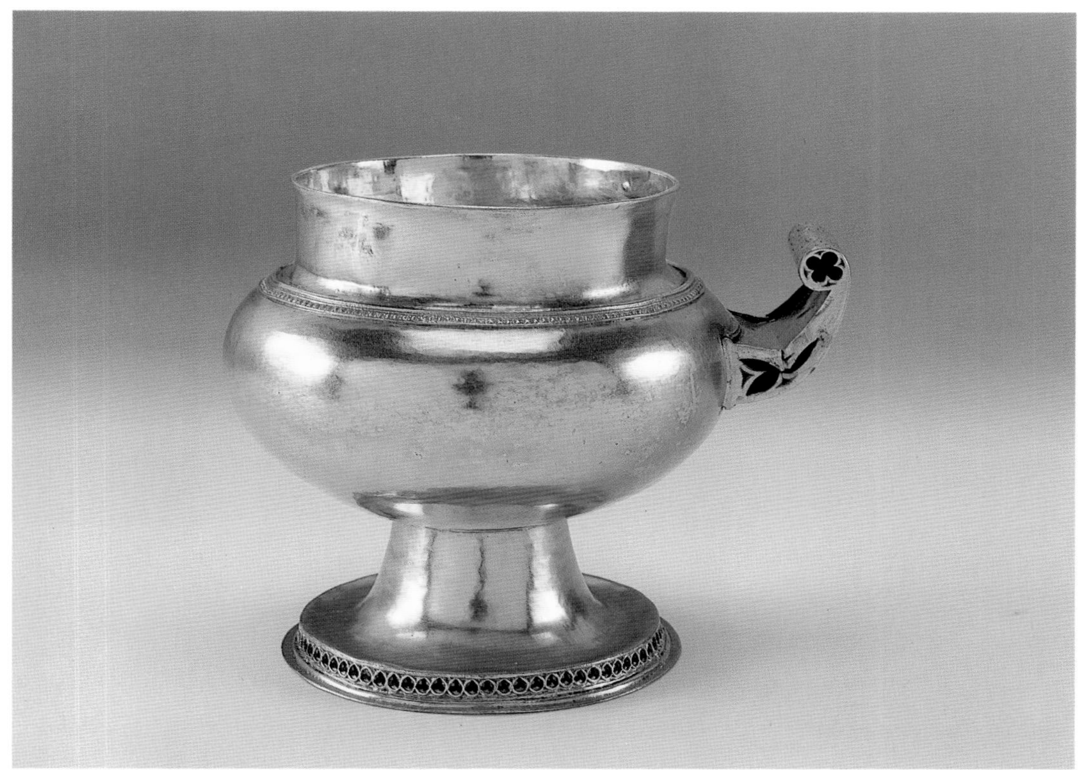

*30*

*31*

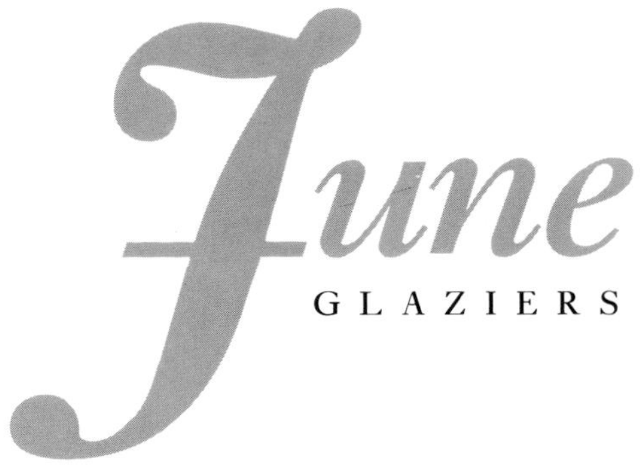

# June
## GLAZIERS

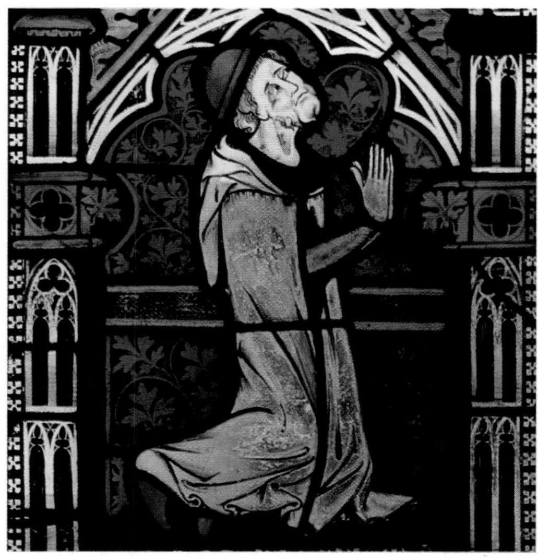

THE STAINED glass windows of the great Gothic Cathedrals are one of the most admired creations of the Middle Ages. At Chartres, the vast expanses of translucent colour transform the interior and create a lasting impression on the visitor. The aim in medieval churches was to pierce the solid masonry of the wall with ever larger and more decorative windows. One of the largest English stained glass windows is the east window of York Minster. This (23 × 10 metres) was glazed under the direction of John Thornton, a glass painter from Coventry. He was the leader of a team of glaziers who completed the work in only three years (1405–8). The range of payments in the teams of glass painters who completed these large works is illustrated by the accounts for the glazing of St Stephen's Chapel in Westminster in 1351–2. Here master glaziers received 12d a day, ordinary glaziers earned 7d and their assistants 4d.

Although most glass painters were anonymous, an exception is Gerlachus, who can be seen holding his brush and paint pot on a panel from Arnstein in Germany. Most painters were men but there were some women who practised, such as Jeanne la Verrière, who was described in a Parisian tax roll between 1292 and 1313.

Glaziers hardly ever made their own sheets of glass but purchased them from glass makers. White sheet glass was certainly produced in England, but the best coloured glass was imported from the continent. Coloured glass was twice as expensive as white glass in England in the fourteenth century. Yellow stained glass was produced by applying silver nitrate to the exterior surface and firing it in a kiln. Usually different colours were divided by lead strips but sometimes 'jewels' of coloured glass were annealed onto draperies and haloes without the use of leads to produce a very colourful effect.

1

*Left* Henry de Mamesfield, shown as the donor on fourteen windows that he gave to Merton College Chapel, Oxford, in the early fourteenth century.

*Below* A medieval glass house in operation; from an early fifteenth-century manuscript of the travels of St John Mandeville produced in Bohemia.

2

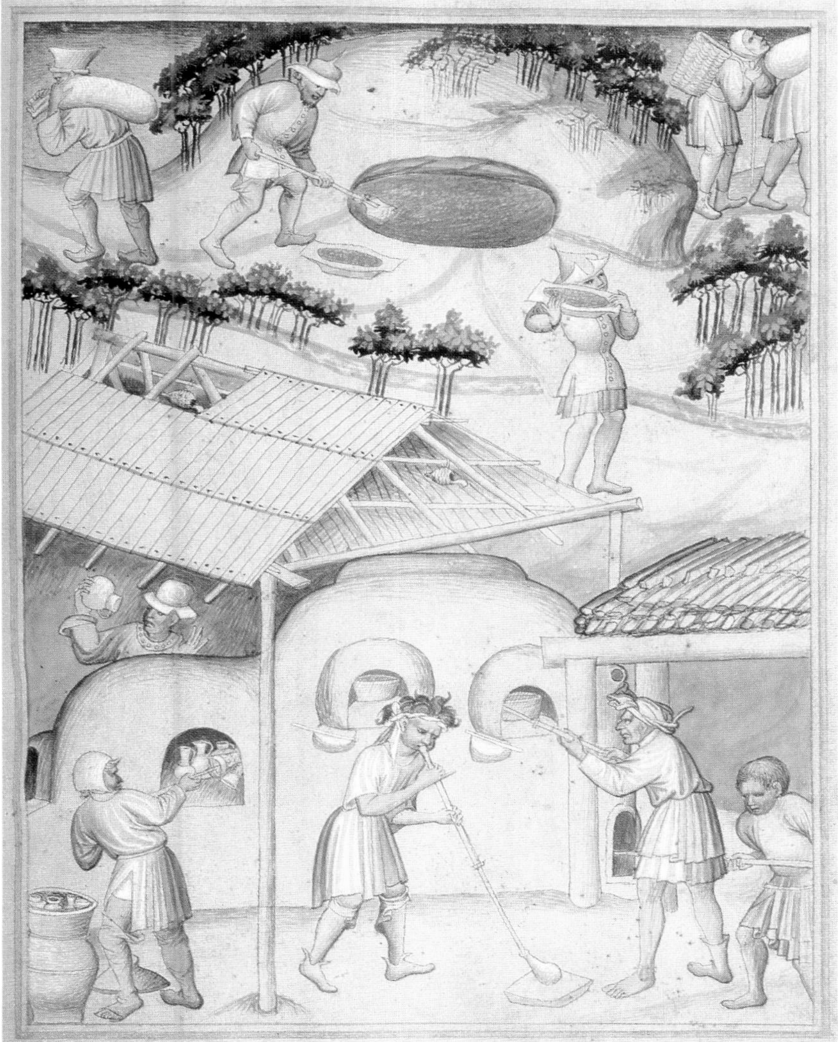

3

4

5

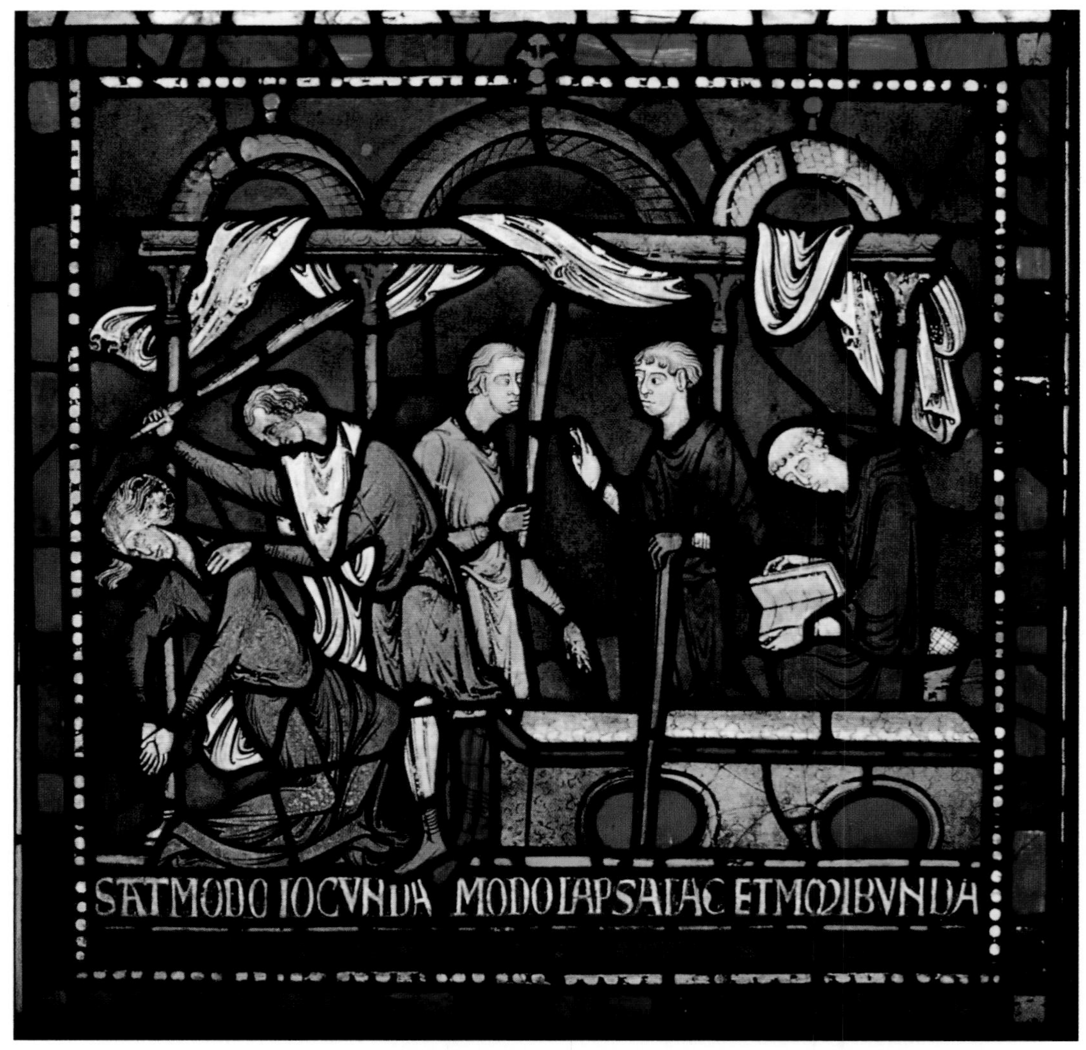


The lady fainting on the left is Mathilda, a mad woman of Cologne, who visited the crypt tomb of St Thomas à Becket at Canterbury. The cure of Mathilda was one of the miracles that the glass painters depicted in the Trinity Chapel of Canterbury Cathedral.

# June

*6*

*7*

*8*

*9*

*10*

*11*

*12*

*13*

*14*

*15*

# June

20

16

21

17

22

18

23

19

24

The Nativity, drawn in 1443, was one of the three scenes commissioned for the *occhi* of Florence Cathedral from the artist Paolo Uccello.

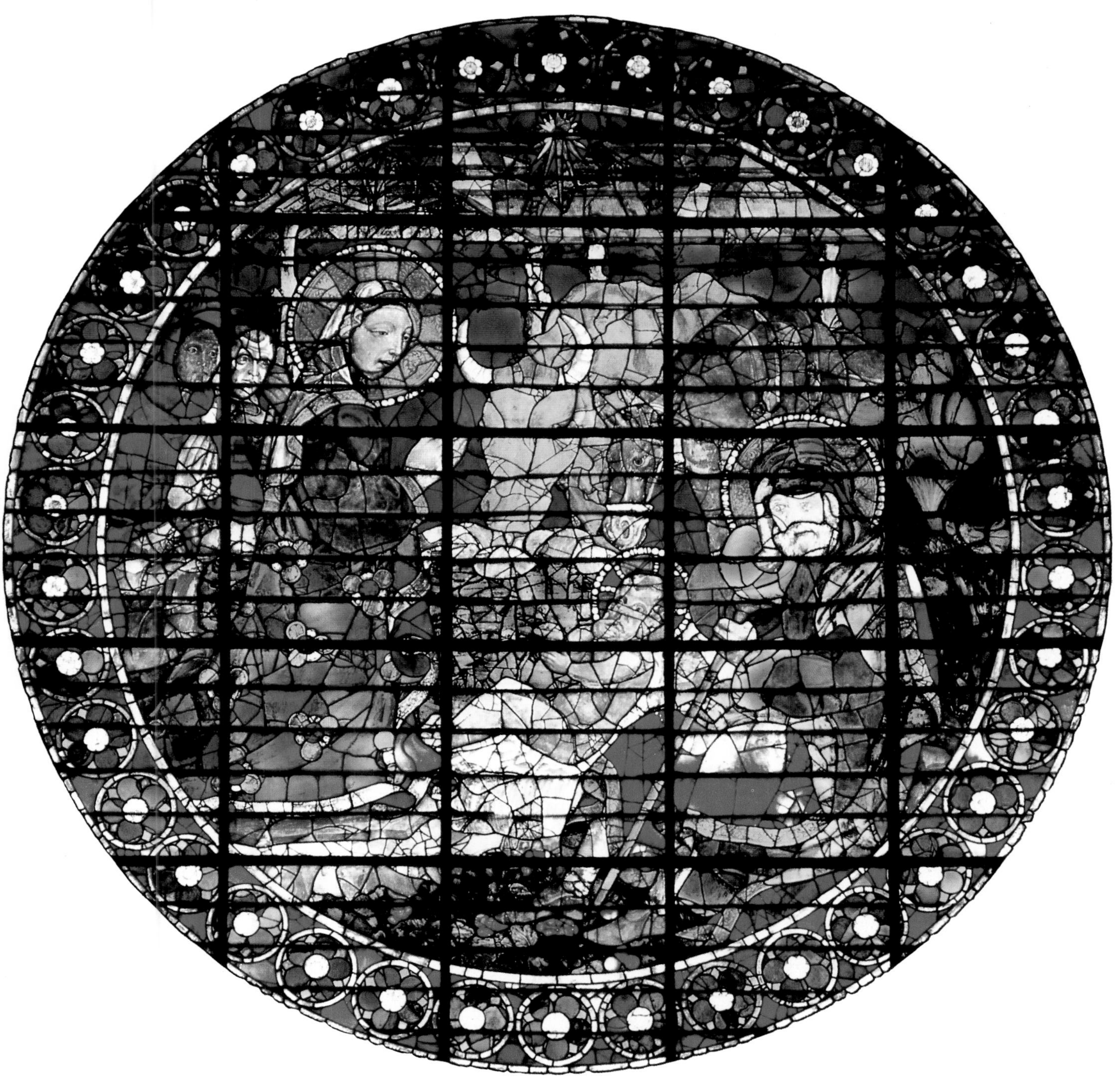

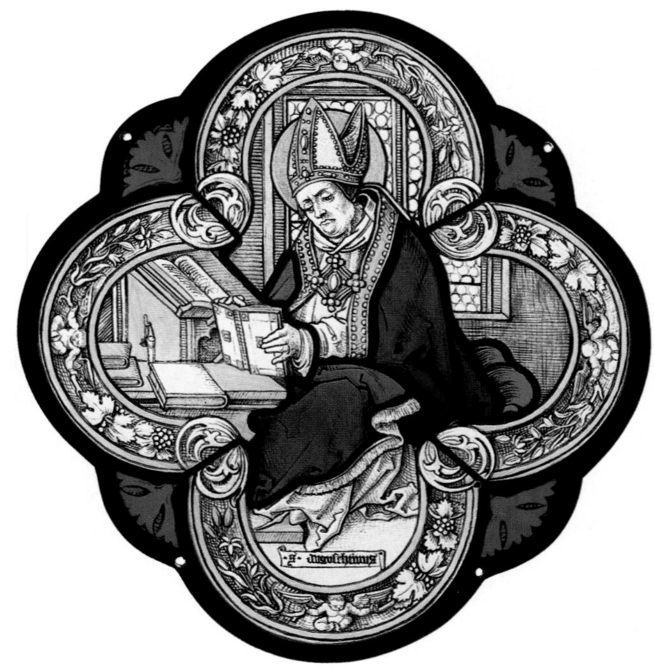

St Augustine of Hippo in his study. The glass panel, painted in the workshop of Veit Hirsvogel the Elder, *c.* 1507, is from an unidentified Nuremberg church.

*Because they are very valuable on account of their wonderful execution and the profuse expenditure of painted glass and sapphire glass, we appointed an official master craftsman for their protection and repair.*

Abbot Suger on his windows at St Denis.

# June

25

26

27

28

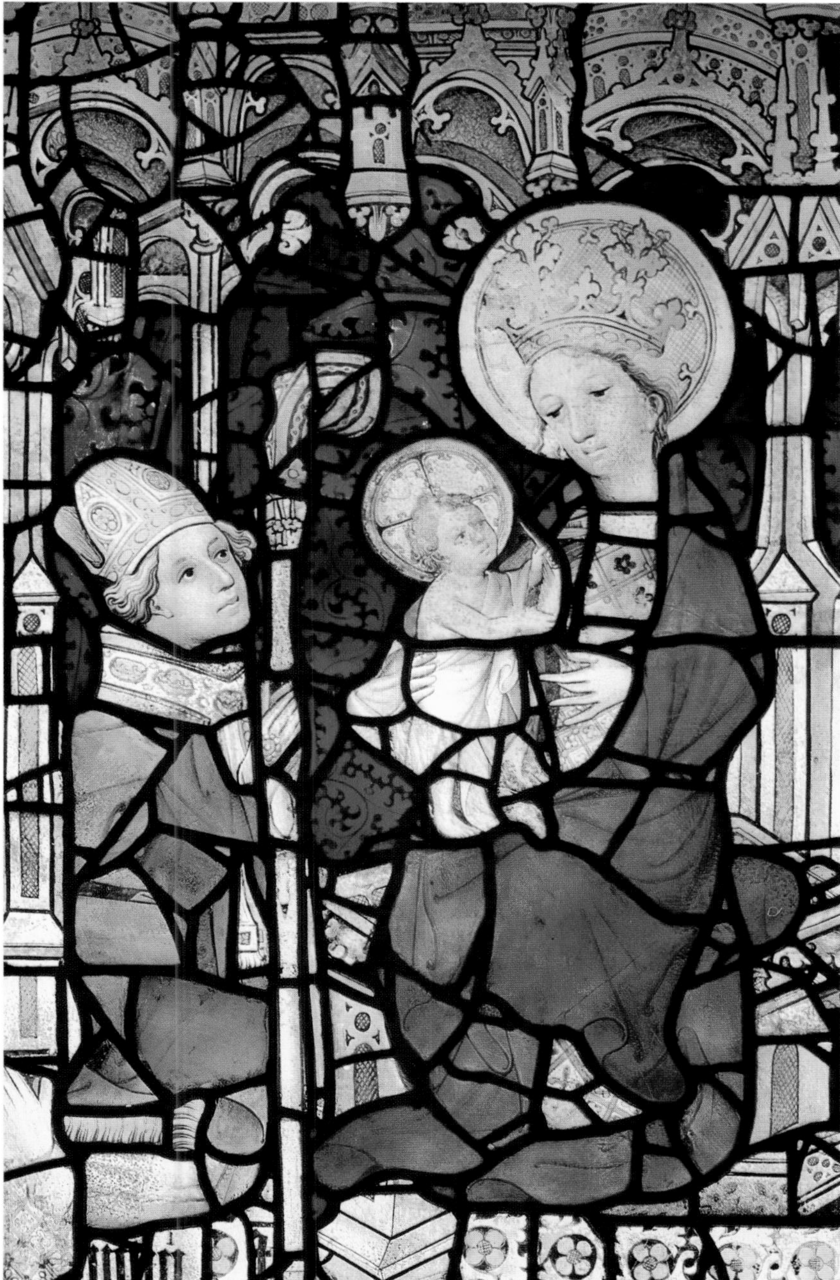

29

30

William of Wykeham is shown kneeling in devotion to the Virgin in a glass panel in Winchester College Chapel. The chapels of his two late fourteenth-century foundations, Winchester College and New College Oxford, were furnished with fine stained glass by the workshop of Thomas Glazier of Oxford.

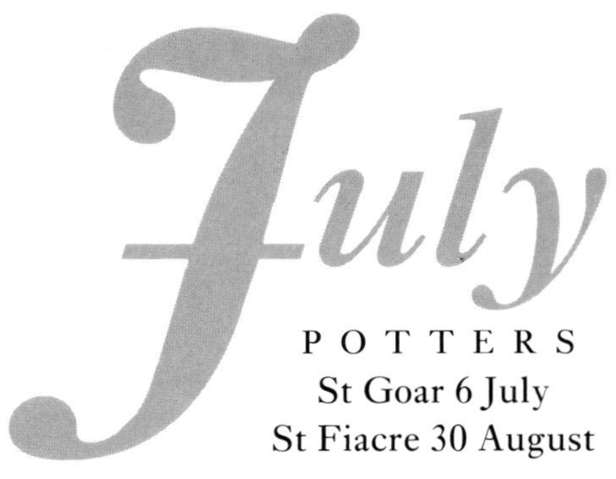

# July

## POTTERS

St Goar 6 July
St Fiacre 30 August

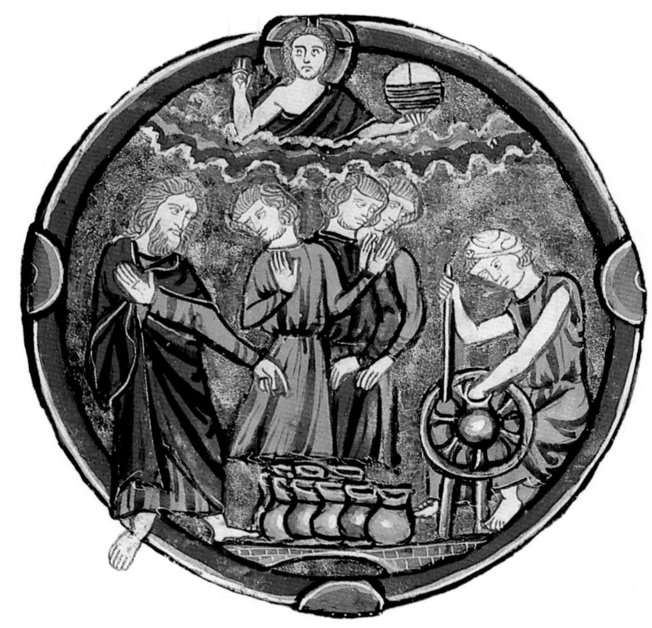

POTTERS WERE among the poorest of the craftsmen. Like tilers they did not have a guild. Nevertheless their products have a remarkable life and vivacity. The jug with brightly coloured green glaze and often boldly formed sculptural decoration is the product for which they are remembered. This craft using clay, a simple material worked with the hands, was perhaps closest to William Morris's later vision of the medieval craftsman.

In the Middle Ages the term 'potter' could mean a craftsman working in either clay or metal and often the correct meaning is only made clear by the context or the price of the goods supplied. In towns the potter probably worked in metal, whilst in villages he is more likely to have used clay. In the country pottery was often pursued as a part-time occupation combined with farming. It was often a subsidiary craft forming part of a web of interwoven rural activity, of which there is little written record. Pottery was often a family concern; at Toynton, in Lincolnshire, sons followed their fathers as potters. Most potters mentioned in documents are men but at Woodstock, in Oxfordshire, Agnes Siber rented a kiln for a penny a year.

Glaze was used decoratively on the outside of jugs. The basic glaze was lead. This was applied with a brush or was sometimes splashed or flicked onto the surface of the vessels. A glaze takes its colour from the body of the pot, so that a pure lead glaze over a pale body produces a yellow colour. The bright green colour was achieved by adding copper filings to the glaze. The depth of colour varies according to the proportion of copper introduced from a yellowish-green to a dark deep even green.

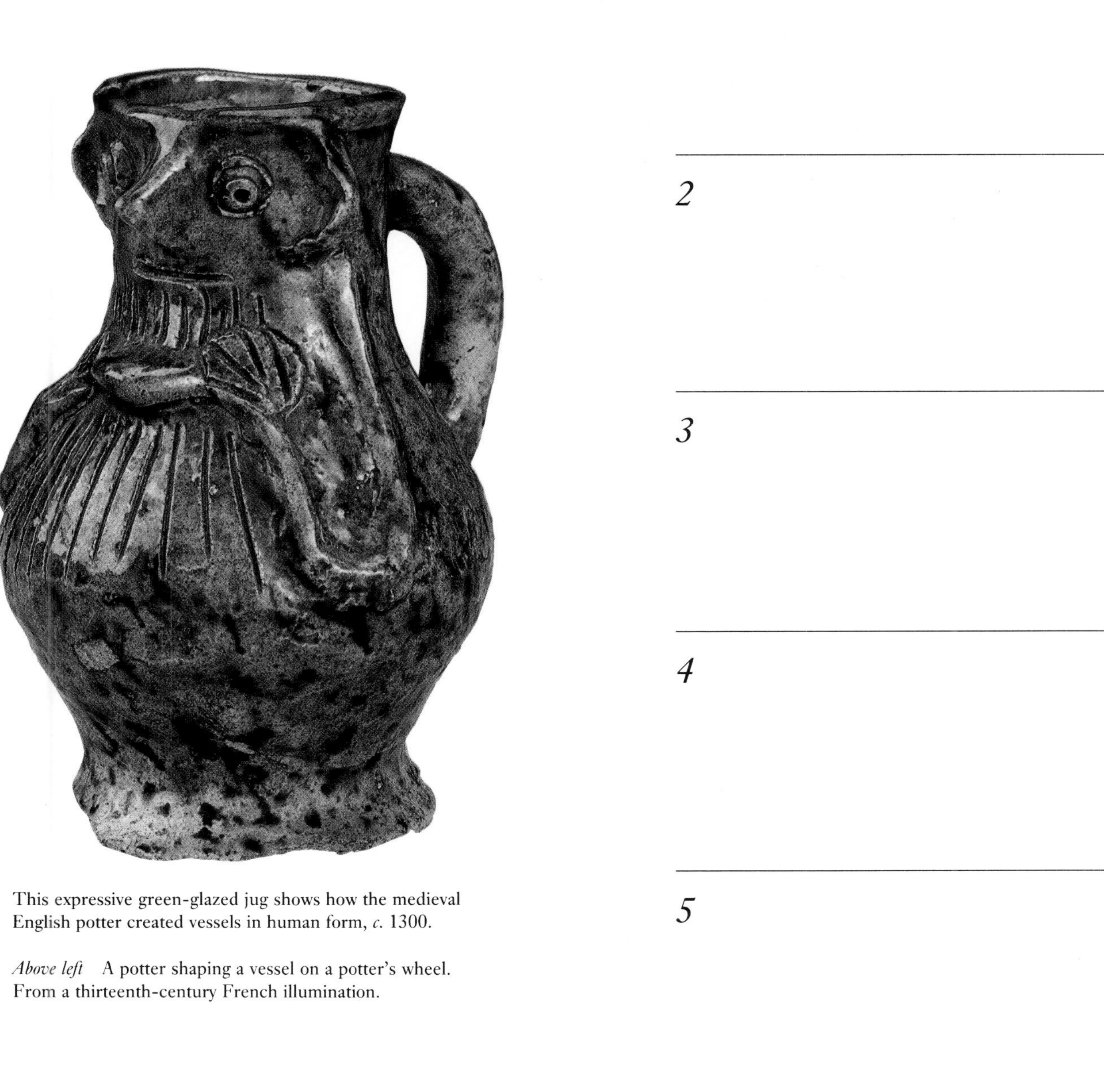

This expressive green-glazed jug shows how the medieval English potter created vessels in human form, *c.* 1300.

*Above left* A potter shaping a vessel on a potter's wheel. From a thirteenth-century French illumination.

*1*

*2*

*3*

*4*

*5*

# July

*My intent is to die in a tavern*
*Where wine is closest to the mouth of the dying;*
*Then the choir of angels will sing more gladly:*
*'May God be propitious to this man of drink.'*
Medieval drinking song.

6

7

8

9

10

11

12

13

14

15

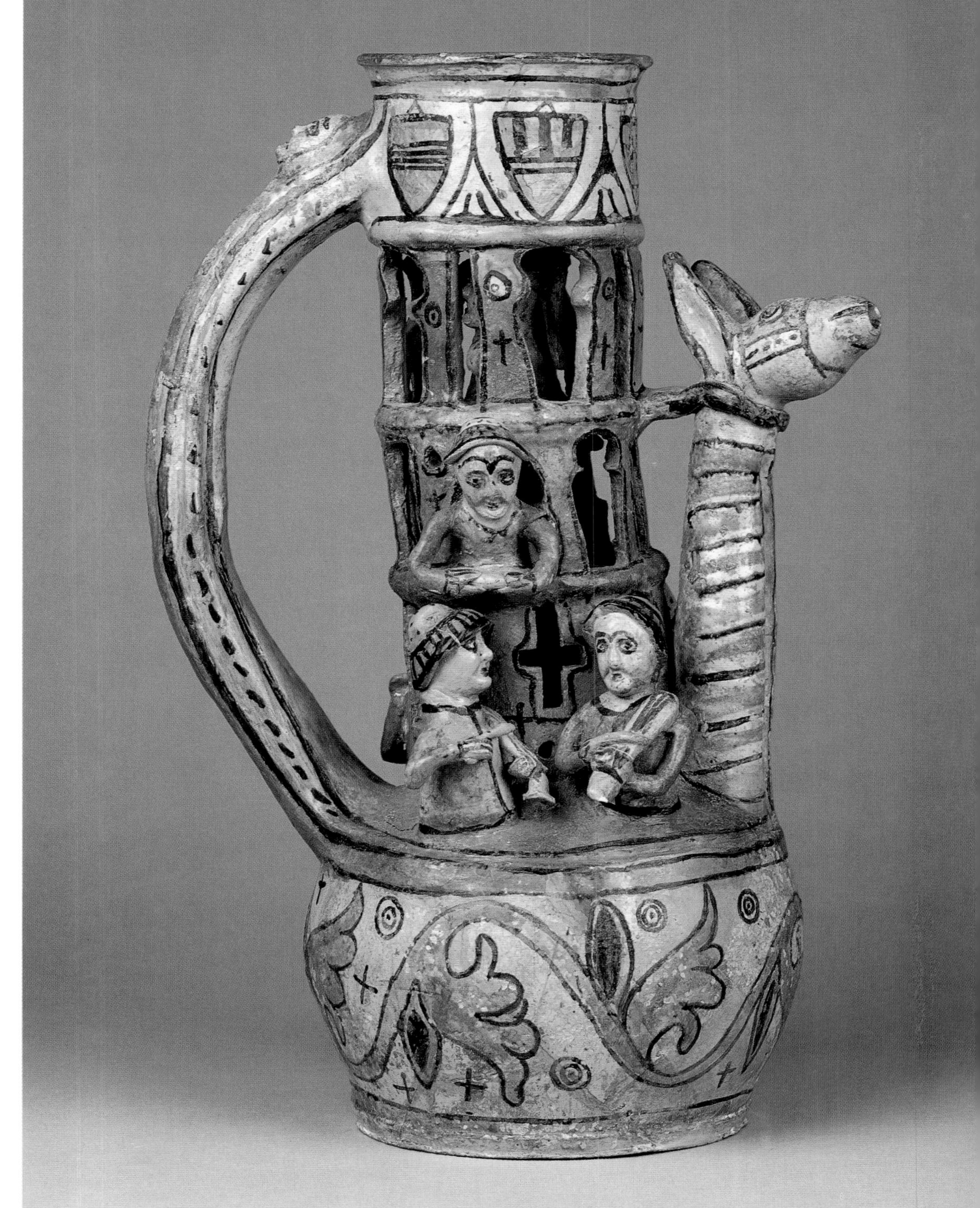

A pottery puzzle jug made in the Saintonge in south-west France *c.* 1300 and found in Exeter, England. The puzzle is that the liquid poured in the top disappears down the hollow handle into the chamber at the bottom to spout forth from the mouth of the animal.

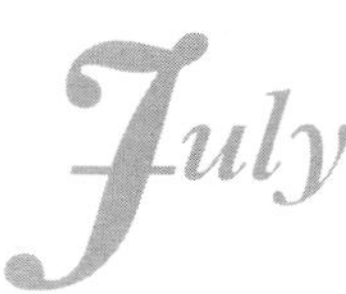

16

17

18

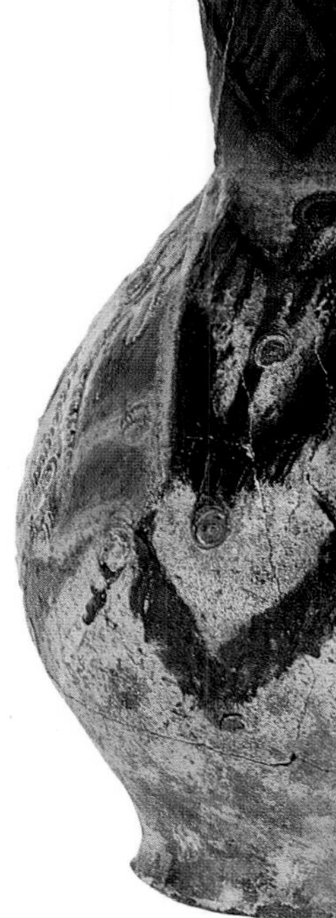

19

20

21

22

*Left* An English pottery jug produced in the thirteenth-century and found in London. The colourful slip decoration of animals in lozenges may indicate that the potter was imitating a French vessel.

*23*

*24*

*25*

*26*

*27*

*28*

*29*

*30*

*31*

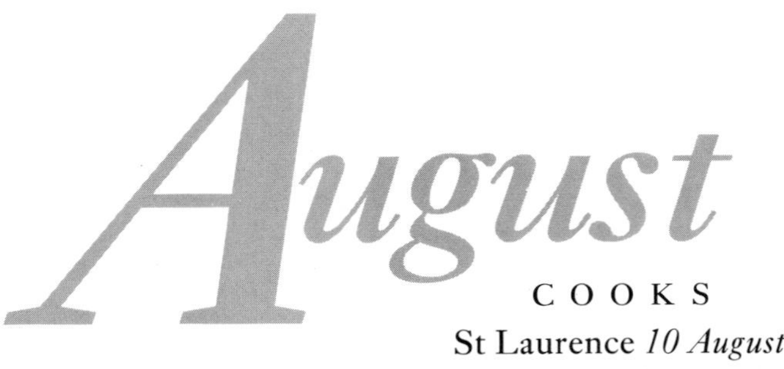


## COOKS

St Laurence *10 August*

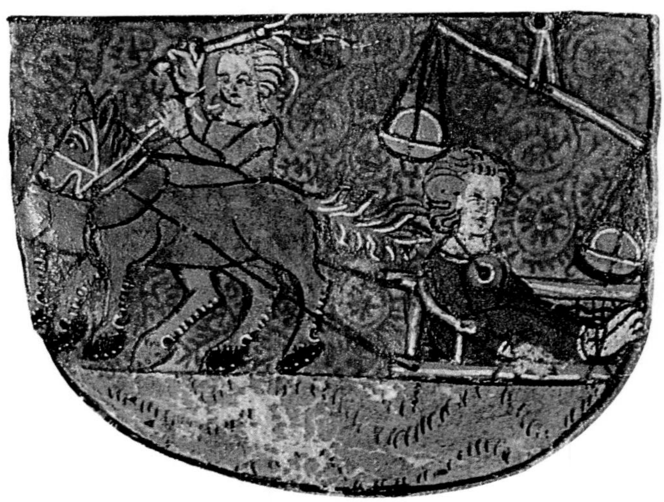

THE COOK in the Middle Ages might be an individual employed in a small household, or a member of a large domestic staff in a big establishment. Alternatively he might work in or even own a tavern or public cooking shop. At such cooking shops cooked meats or pies could be bought to eat at home or customers could bring their own meat to be cooked. The list of prices fixed by the City of London authorities in 1378 includes pig, duck, goose and many other kinds of bird. The most expensive roast meats were best roast bittern at 20d each, heron at 18d each and pheasant at 13d, while the cheapest were ten finches for 1d. The best capon baked in a pasty cost 8d. Regulations in London forbade cooks and piemen to use offal as a filling for pies and to cook meat twice for sale, both of which were very sensible provisions.

King Richard II (1377–99) was particularly interested in fine cooking and in finding new combinations of contrasting flavours. In his reign his master cook compiled the cookery book entitled *The Forme of Cury*. In the prologue Richard is accounted ‘the best and ryallest vyander of all Christian Kings’. The book consists of 196 recipes, many of which use considerable amounts of spices such as ginger, pepper, nutmeg and saffron.

The name of the author is unknown, but we do know the names of two other of Richard’s master cooks. Master Thomas Beauchef became an emeritus cook in 1383 due to old age. He was succeeded by John Goodrich, who had been in the royal kitchens from 1363, and who remained there until 1393. The name of another cook, Master John Brodeye, is preserved because he created an intricate castle to decorate the royal table at the wedding of Edward I’s daughter, Margaret, in 1290.

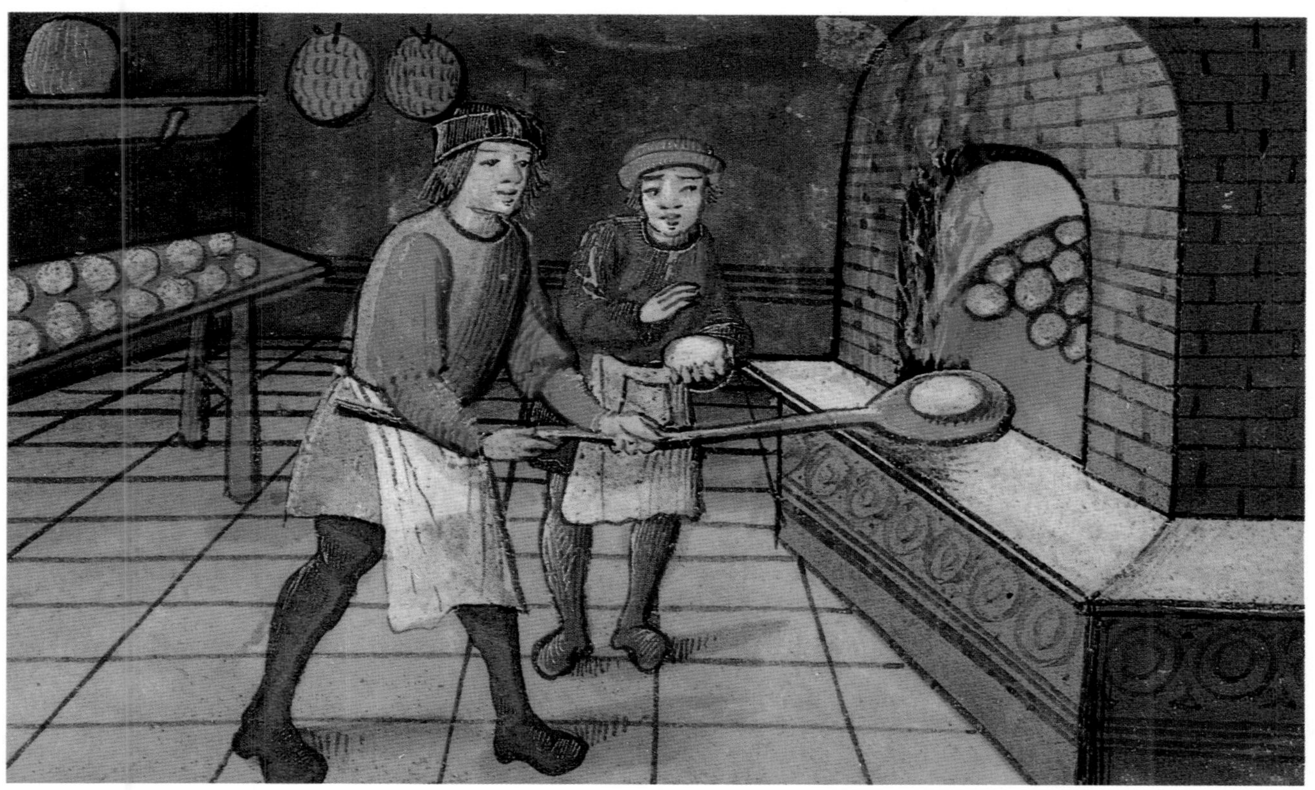

*Above left* A baker who gave short weight is dragged through the streets on a sledge with the offending loaf round his neck.

*Above* A baker and his assistant at work at the oven. They are baking a large batch of fine white bread rolls.

1

2

3

4

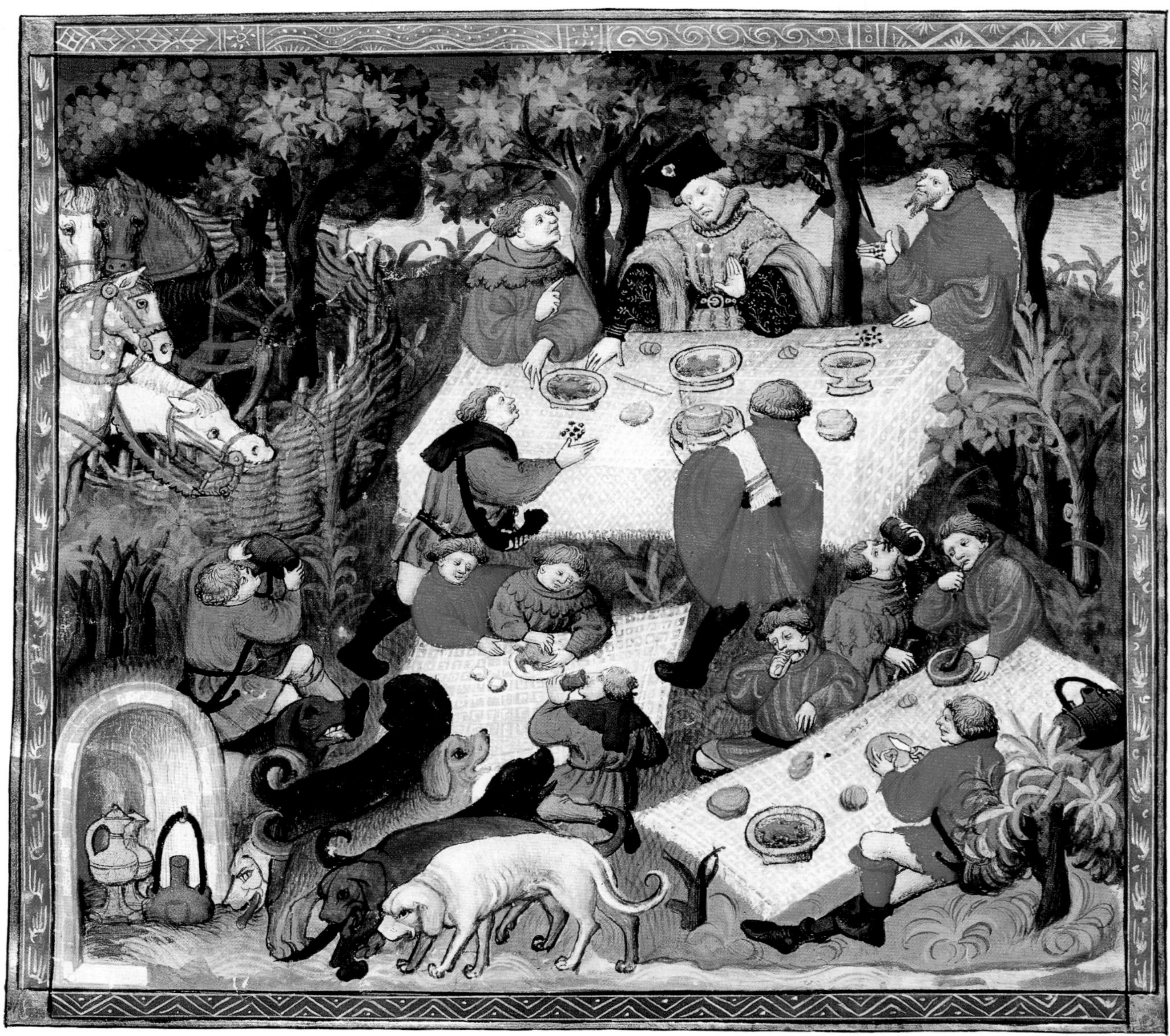

A hunting party stops for the midday meal. Social hierarchy is carefully observed. The lord and his companions are seated at a separate table from the huntsmen who are themselves seated above the dogs.

# August

5

6

7

8

9

10

11

12

13

14

# August

15

20

16

21

17

22

18

23

19

24

*Tourteletes in Frytour. Take figus and grynde hem smal; do therin saffron and powder fort. Close hem in foyles of dowe, and frye hem in oyle. Clarifye hony and flamme hem therwyt; ete hem hote or colde.*

Recipe for fried fig pastries.

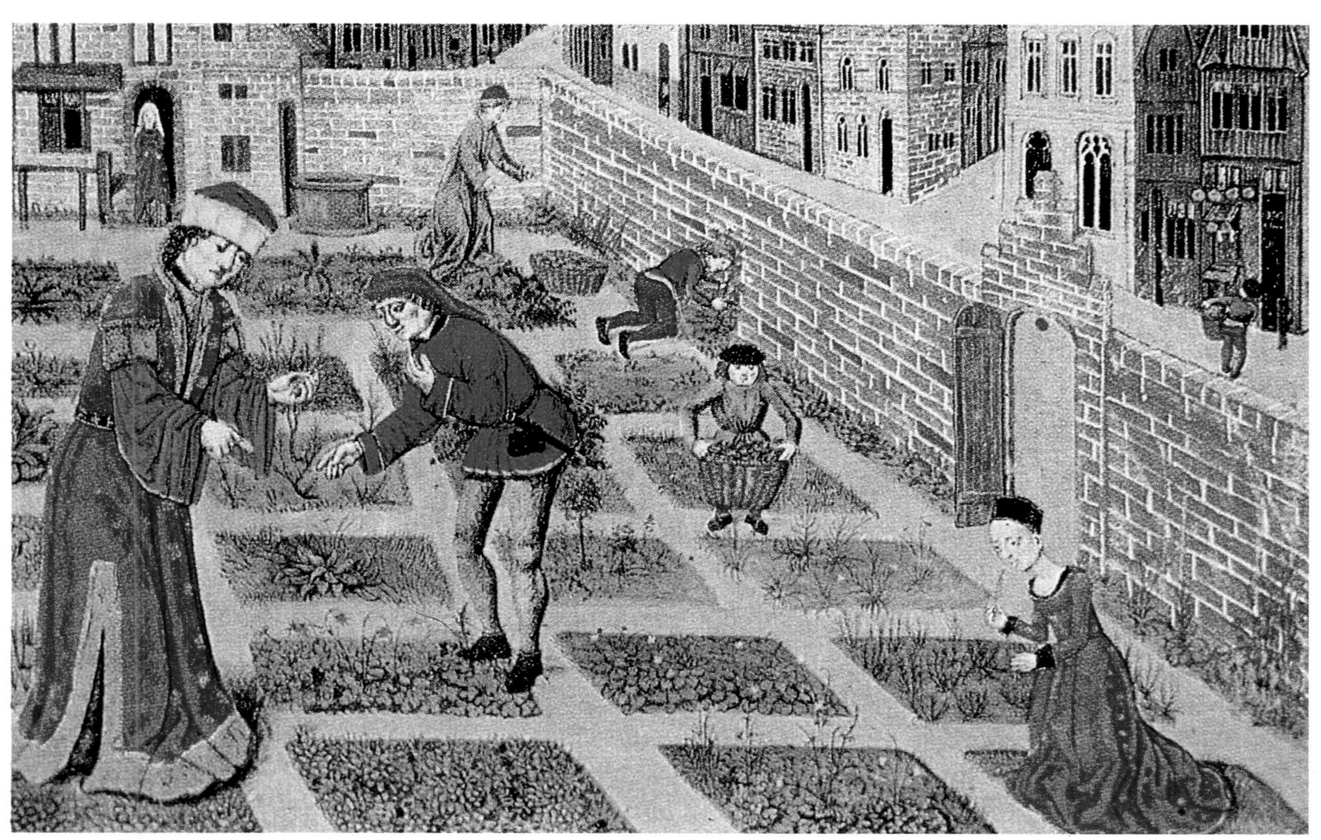

The walled herb garden is divided by paths into rectangular plots, from which assorted herbs are being gathered for kitchen use.

# August

25

26

27

28

29

30

31

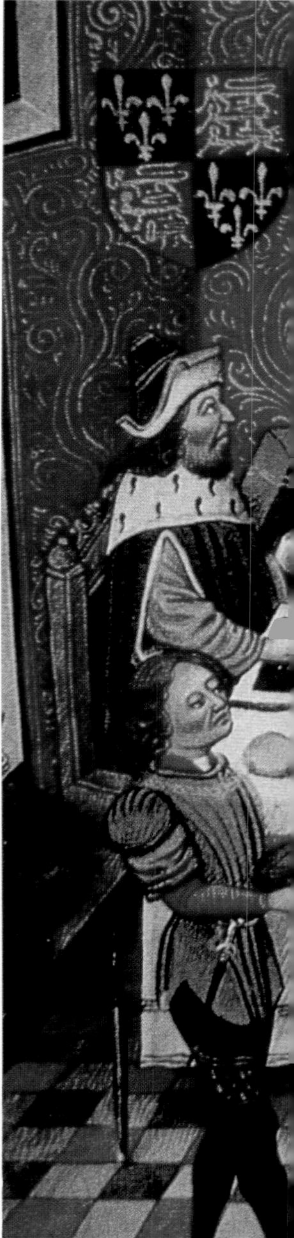

John of Gaunt dines with two kings and four bishops. The serving men bring the cooked food from the kitchen. The illumination shows how the table would be set for such a feast.

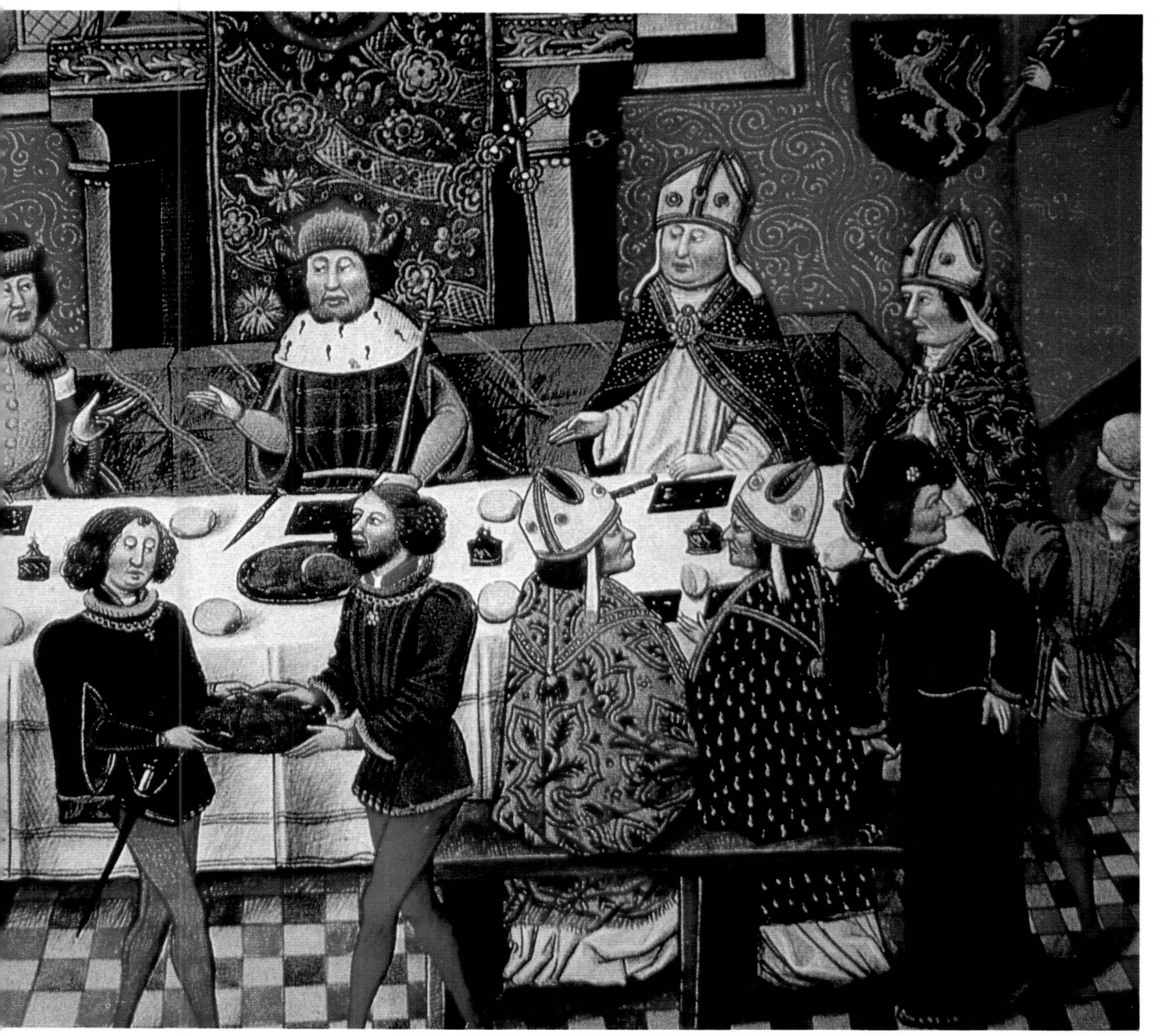

# September

TILERS

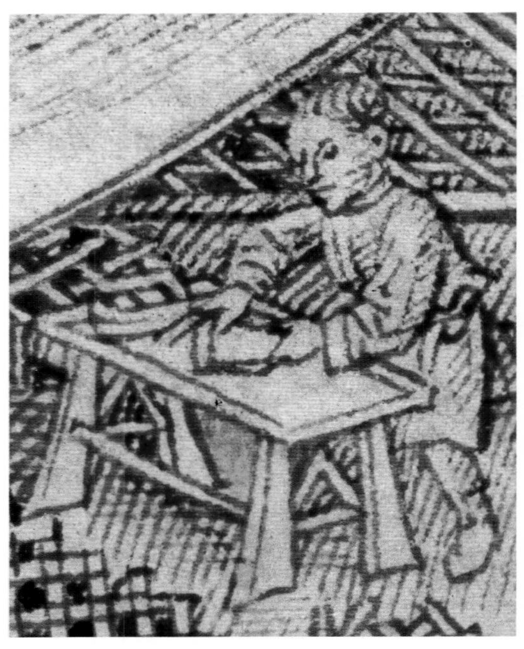

TILERS PRODUCED roofing tiles as well as decorated and plain floor tiles. It is often difficult to know whether the word tiler in medieval documents applies to those craftsmen who actually made roof or floor tiles or to those who positioned them. In the tenth century, decorated floor tiles were made for monastic houses at Winchester, St Albans and Bury St Edmunds. These were probably made by monastic tilers. As late as the thirteenth century, some of the monks in Cistercian monasteries may have taken part in the manufacture of elaborate tile mosaic.

The highly decorated, two-coloured floor tile, which is the most characteristic product of the medieval tiler, was introduced into England in the mid-thirteenth century. At first these tiles appeared in Cistercian abbeys and royal palaces. It seems certain that the tiler making the decorated tiles for the King's Chapel at Clarendon Palace in the mid-thirteenth century had already been working at Beaulieu Abbey and at St Denys Priory in Southampton. Commercial tileries were operating during the later thirteenth century. Commercial tilers usually made a far greater number of tiles from the same amount of clay and they gradually reduced the depth of the expensive white clay that was either inlaid into the tile or painted on as slip.

Some of the most expensive and unusual medieval tiles with elaborate decoration are the series associated with Tring church in Hertfordshire. They illustrate scenes from the infancy miracles of Christ. The pictures closely resemble those in an illuminated manuscript still preserved in the Bodleian Library in Oxford. It is likely that cartoons were made for the tilers to copy since no manuscript would have been allowed anywhere near the messy sand and clay of the tilery.

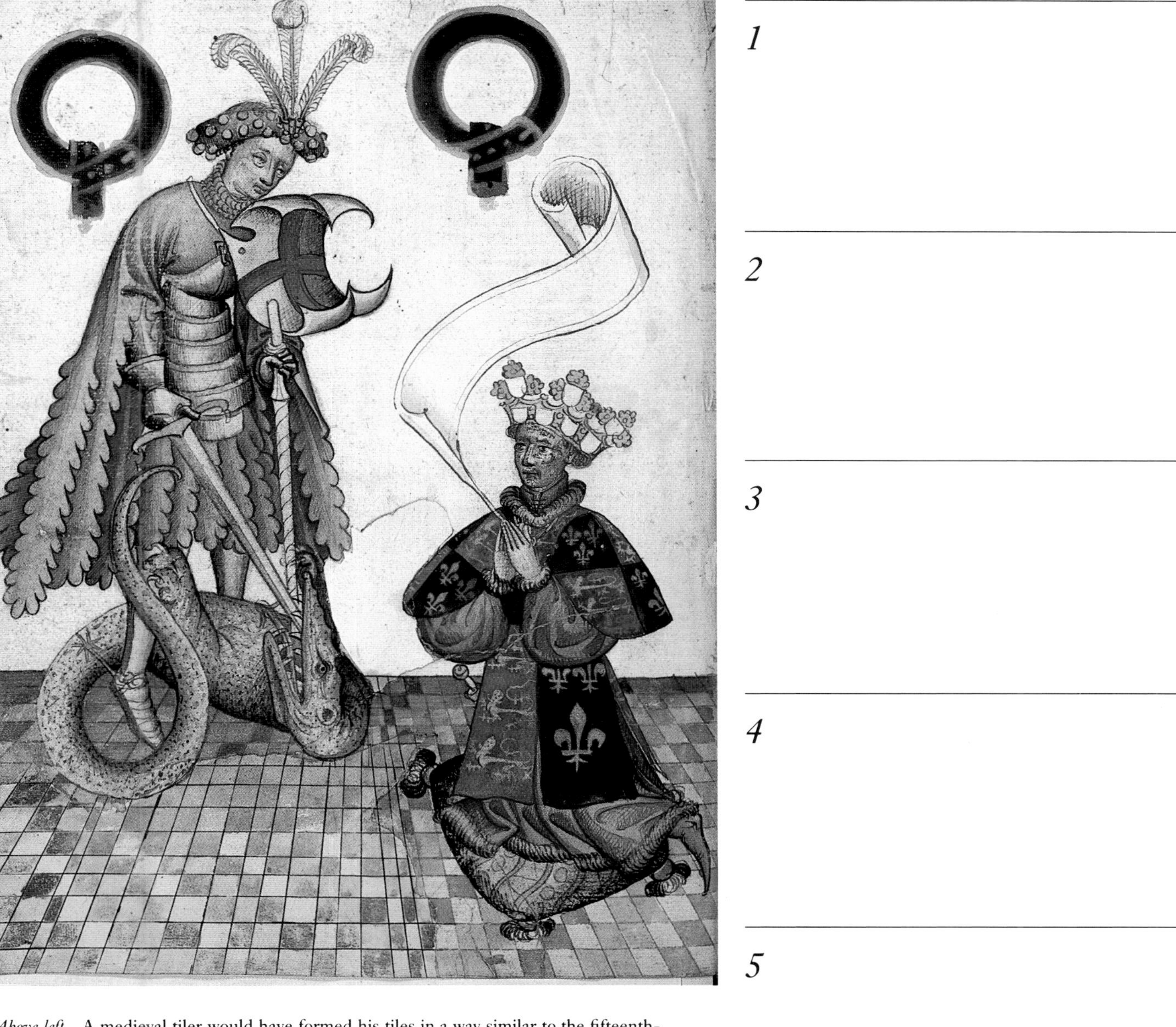

*Above left* A medieval tiler would have formed his tiles in a way similar to the fifteenth-century brickmaker shown above.

*Above* Pavement of plain glazed tiles in different colours on which William Bruges, first Garter King of Arms, kneels before St George. Fifteenth century.

*1*

*2*

*3*

*4*

*5*

# September

*Think, man, thy life may not ever endure,*
*What thou dost thyself, of that thou art sure;*
*But that thou keepest unto thy executor's cure,*
*An ever it avail thee, it is but aventure.*

Inscription on a tile in Malvern Abbey urging the reader not to defer what he might do today.

*6*

*7*

*8*

*9*

*10*

*11*

*12*

*13*

*14*

*15*

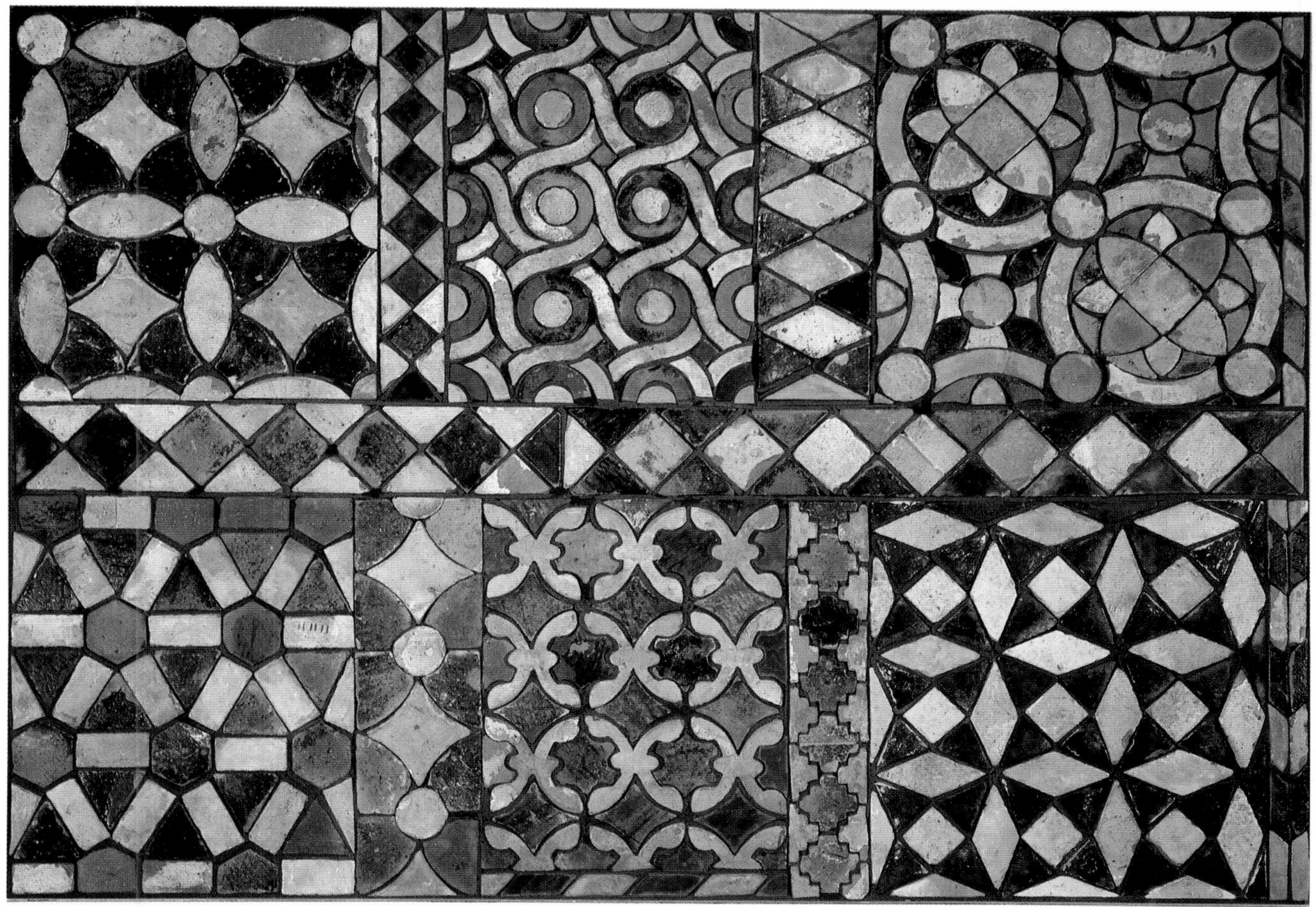

Panel assembled in the British Museum using loose tiles of the mid-thirteenth century from Rievaulx Abbey, Yorkshire. It shows a variety of the panel and border arrangements that the mosaic tile-makers had used there.

*Overleaf* Relief decorated tiles made at the commercial tilery of Bawsey, Norfolk, in the late fourteenth century. The designs are a mixture of heraldry and inscriptions including the name THOMAS (in reverse!).

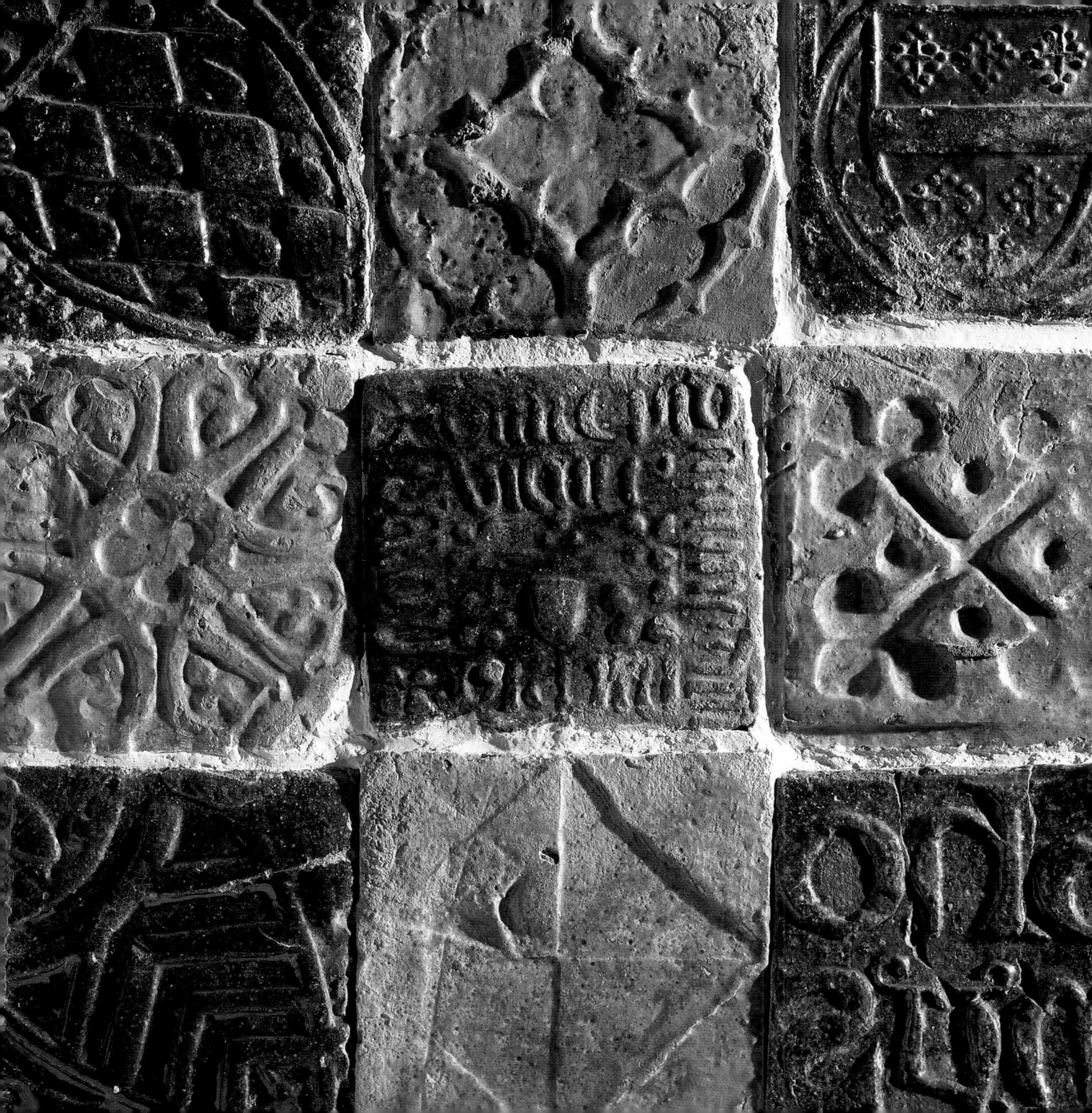

# September

16

17

18

19

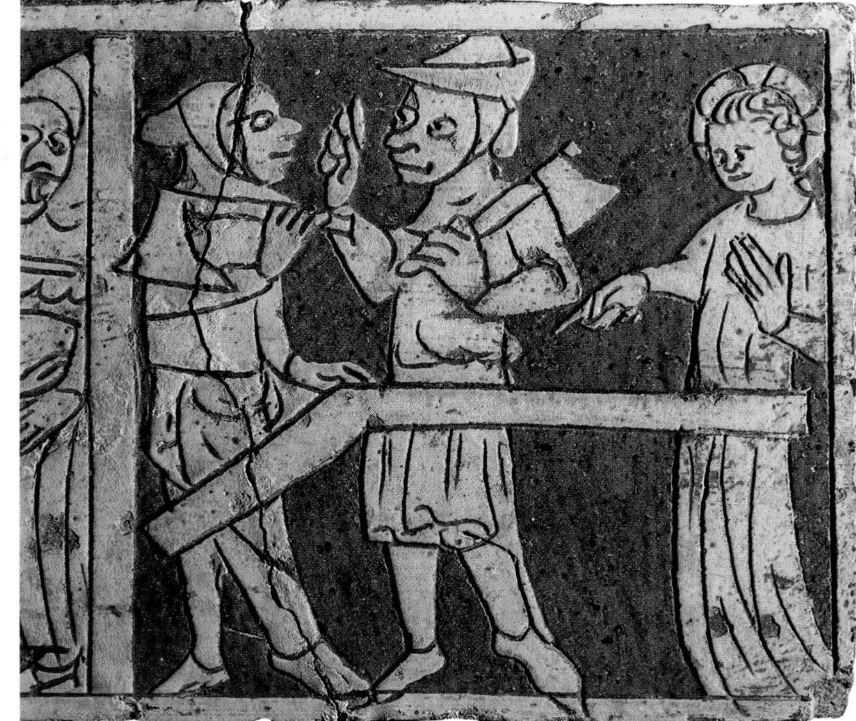

20

21

*Above* The child Jesus points to a broken plough beam which he is about to straighten in a miracle. This early fourteenth-century tile, decorated with lines incised through the slip, is one of a series from Tring church, Hertfordshire.

# September

22

23

24

25

26

27

28

29

30

*Right* Segment of a circular pavement made for the new chapel of Henry III, built in the 1240s, at Clarendon Palace, Wiltshire. This arrangement was assembled from loose tiles recovered during the excavations.

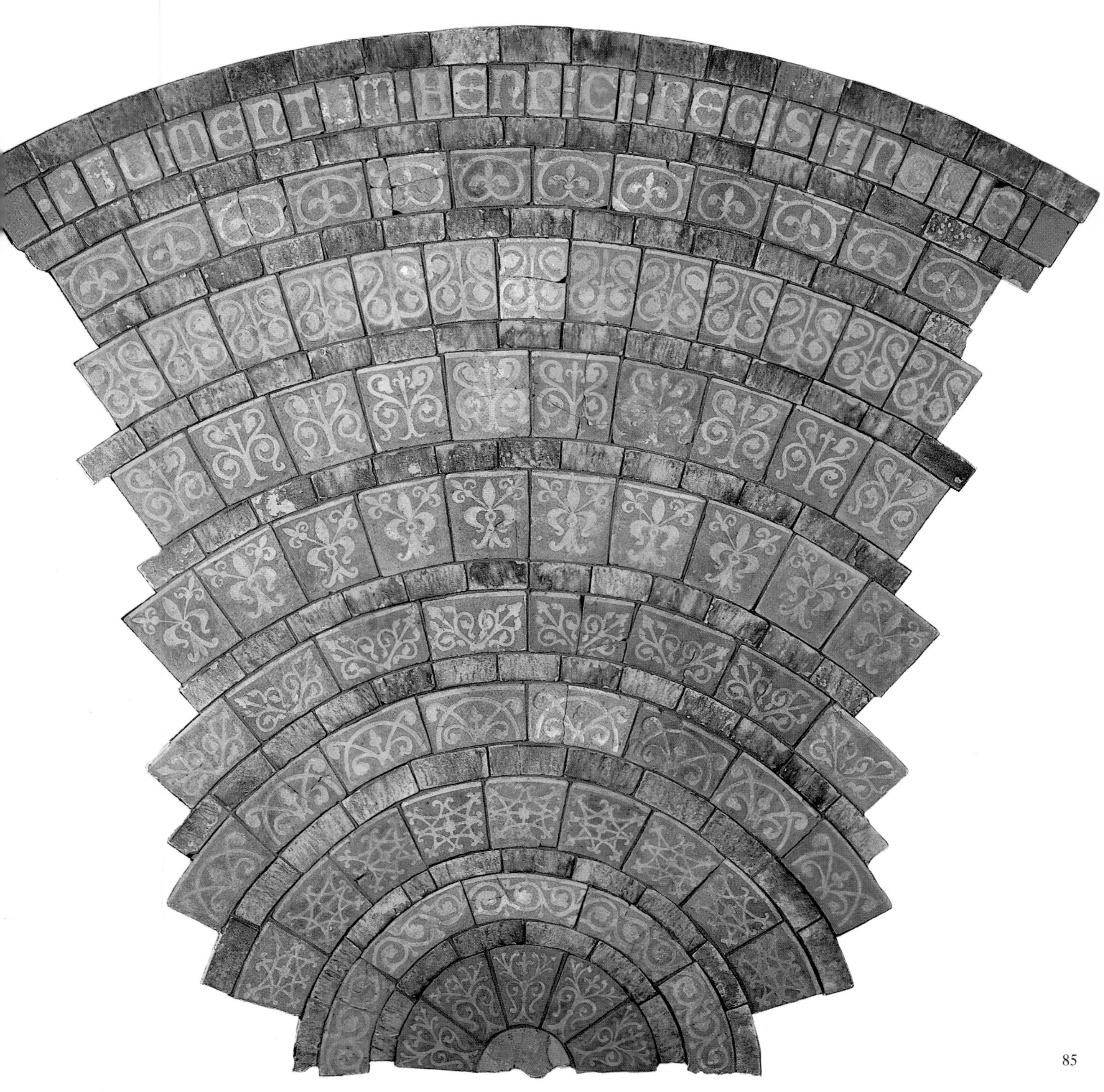

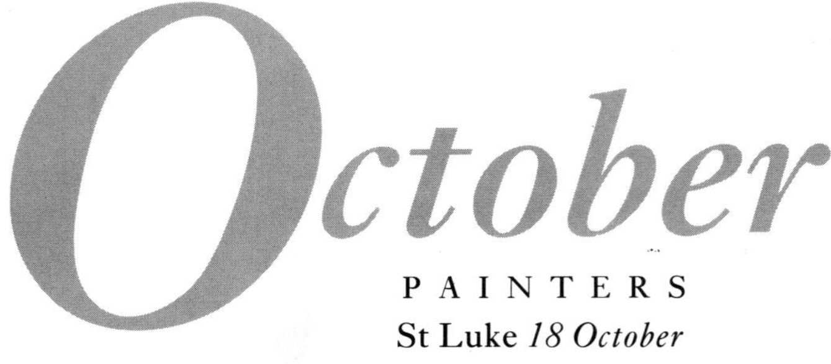

# October

PAINTERS

St Luke *18 October*

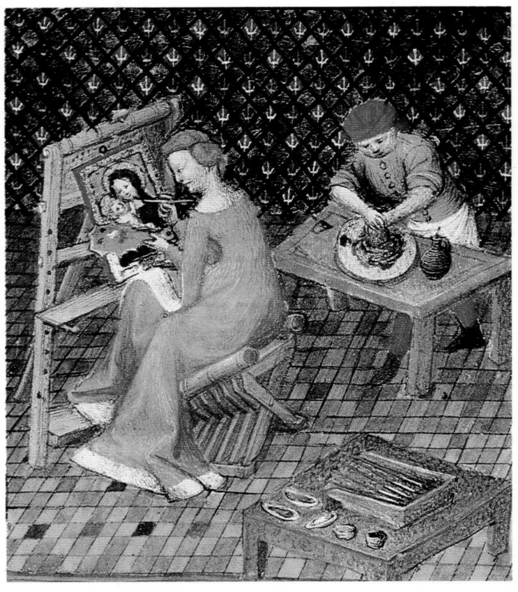

WHILE ILLUMINATORS decorated vellum with paint and gold leaf, painters coloured plastered walls or wooden panels. Some painters, particularly in the eleventh to thirteenth centuries, were monks. While some painters may have worked solely within their monastery or order, others travelled widely, such as William, a Benedictine monk of Westminster, who painted for King Henry III (1216–72) in Winchester, Westminster and Windsor. The painters' guilds had great influence in the fourteenth and fifteenth centuries. The painter would usually have an apprenticeship of four to eight years. Some painters eventually qualified as a Master (Magister) by presenting a masterpiece to the guild.

There is very little evidence that women painted panels or walls. Some female participation is mentioned, mainly as helpers who prepared and fetched materials. This contrasts with the portrayal of famous antique lady painters in Boccaccio's book, *On famous women*, where the ladies are painting, whilst a male assistant prepares the colours. But this is real life turned upside down.

In some secular painting the patrons often dictated the images to be produced by the painters. The noble lady, Mahaut, Countess of Artois, gave clear instructions for the paintings of her father's crusading exploits in her residence in the early fourteenth century. They included a scene of the count throwing two barrels of wine into a fountain, around which inscriptions were to explain the story succinctly. Religious images were more often controlled by a traditional sense of what was customary and proper. One of the finest examples of a religious wall painting scheme, which is both didactic and very moving, is that in the Arena Chapel, Padua, painted by Giotto in 1305. Medieval visitors not only saw the paintings, but by doing so also obtained relief from their time in Purgatory.

*Left* The lady paints while the man grinds her colours, from a French copy made in 1402 of Boccacio's *De claris mulieribus (On famous women).*

*Below* The initial C from *Omne Bonum*, the earliest alphabetical encyclopedia. English *c.* 1350. This shows colour as a series of painters' dishes.

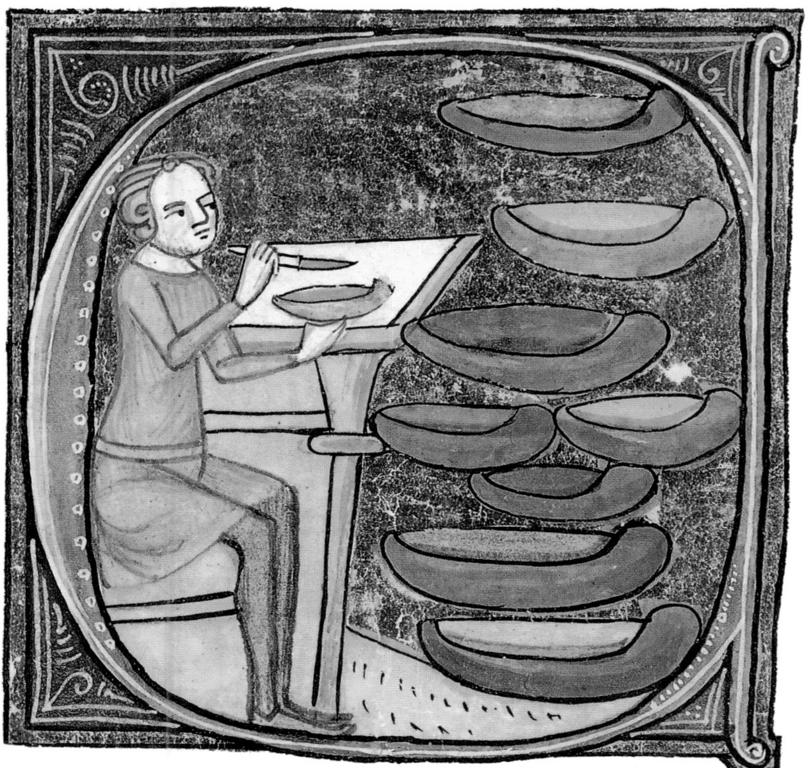

*1*

*2*

*3*

*4*

*5*

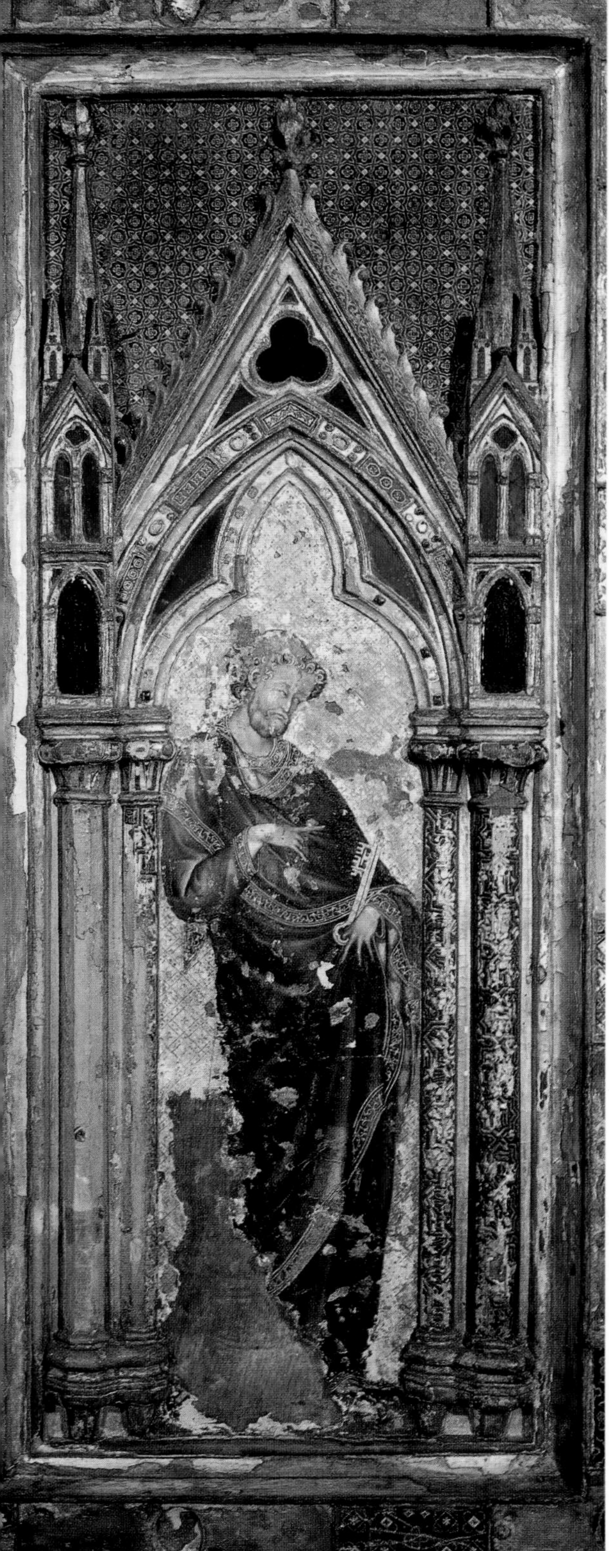

# October

*He had such skills in the working of gold and silver and other metal, and in painting pictures, that it is thought that there has been none to equal him in the Latin world.*
Praise of the St Albans monk, Matthew Paris.

St Peter, from the Westminster Retable, Westminster Abbey, late thirteenth century. One of the most decoratively complex altarpieces in existence, the paintings are executed in linseed oil and the minutely-carved oak frame is set with glass plaques, jewel-like beads, paste cameos and imitation enamels.

*6*

*7*

*8*

*9*

*10*

*11*

*12*

*13*

*14*

*15*

*16*

*17*

An early representation of St Luke as a painter, *c.* 1360, executed in Bohemia in the *Gospel Book of John of Troppau*. Note the brush-rest, and the addition by St Luke of a thin undercoat to the panel sketch of the Crucifixion.

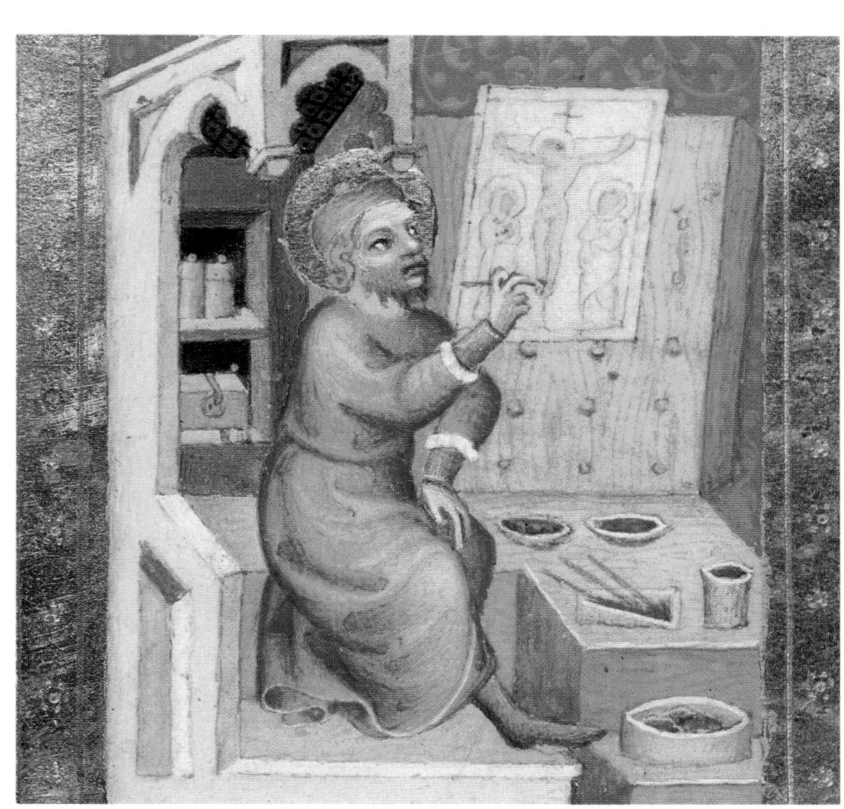

# October

*18*

*19*

*20*

*21*

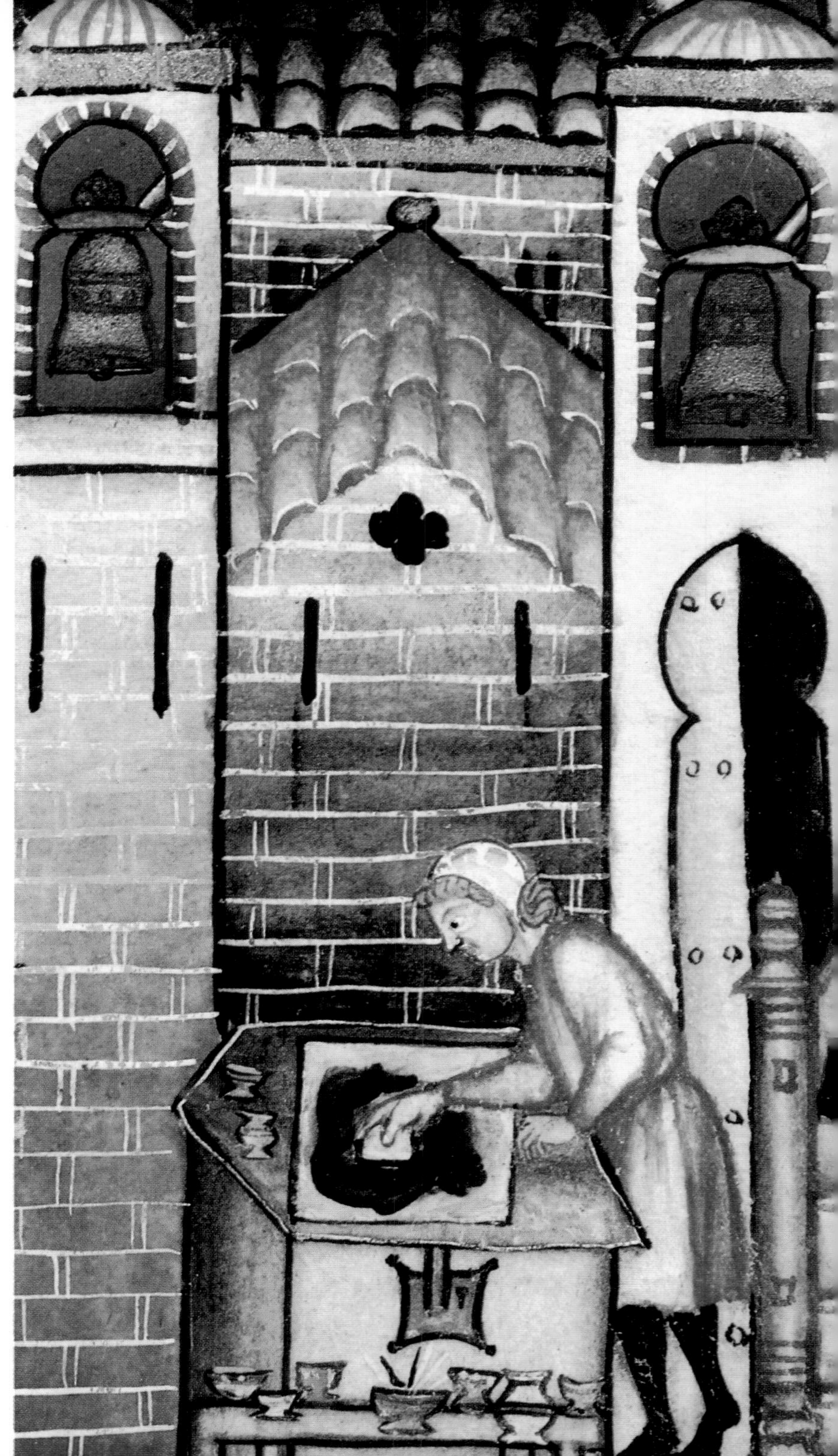

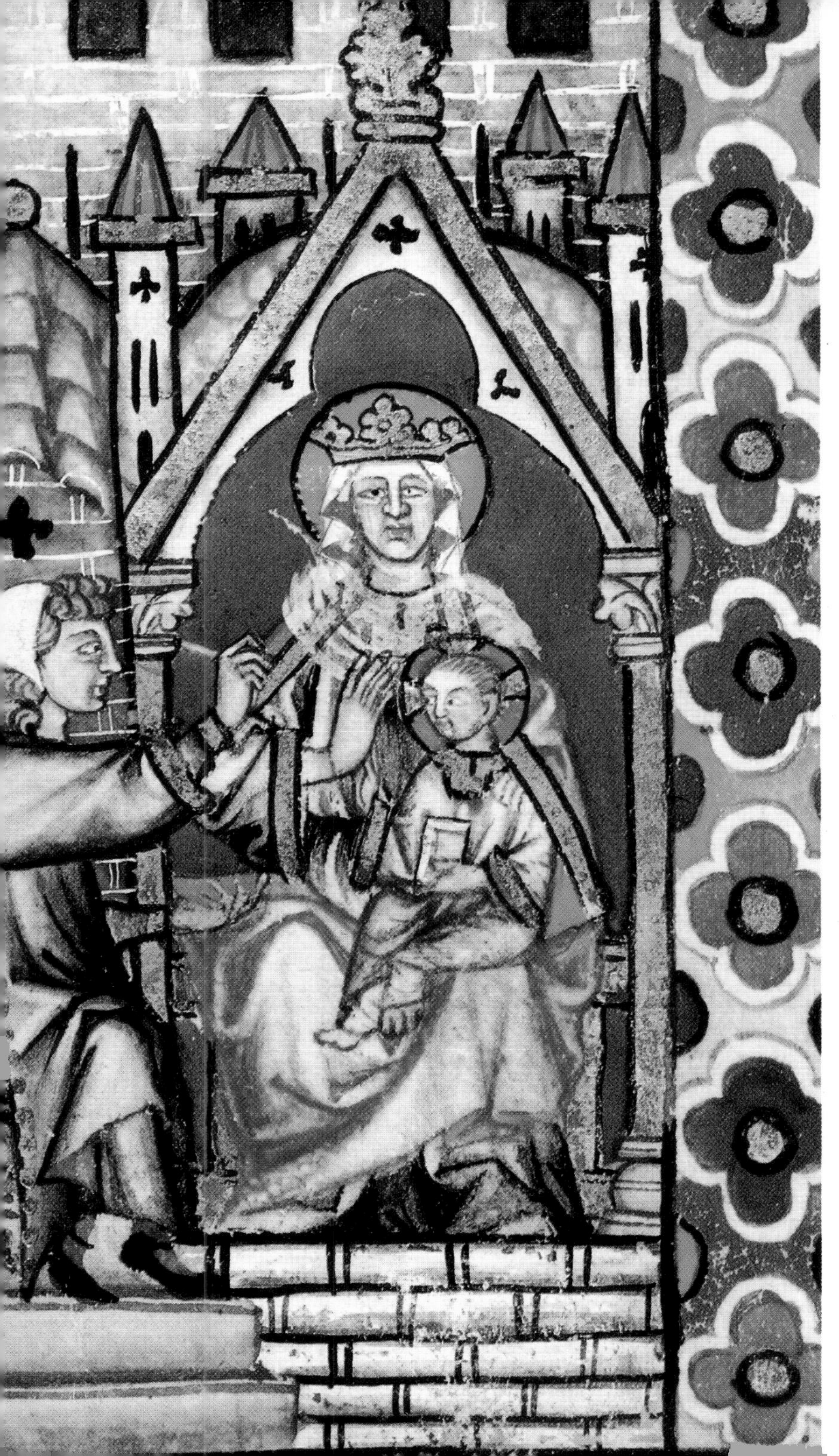

22

23

24

25

26

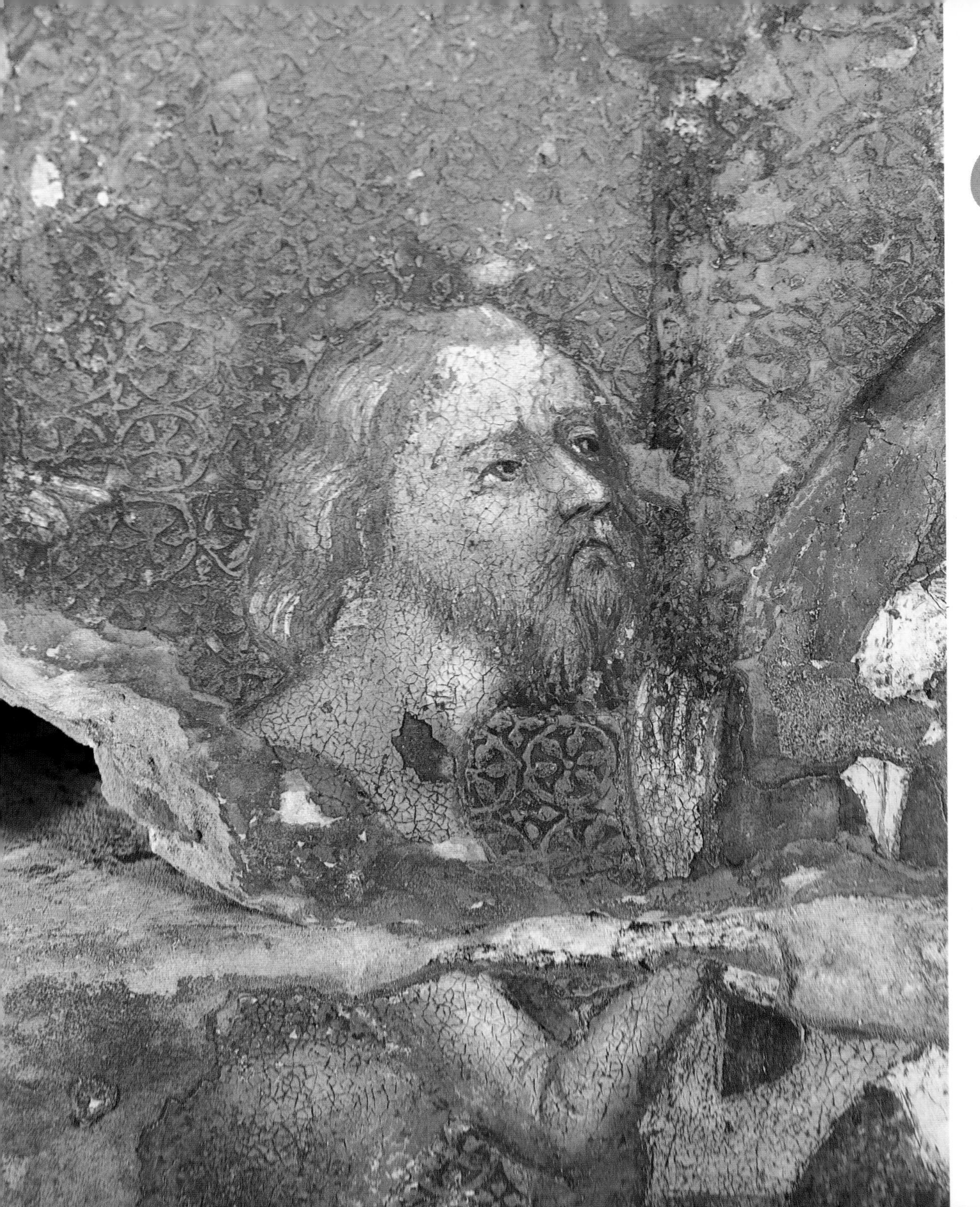

# October

*Previous pages* Painters at work on a carved image of the Virgin Mary; to the left, colours are ground on a block. From *Las Cantigas* of King Alphonso the Wise of Castile, late thirteenth century.

*Left* Job, a detail from the St Stephen's Chapel murals, formerly in Westminster Palace, *c.* 1350–60. The ground has been treated with embossed red lead, from which the gilding has worn off. The medium is oil paint, similar to a panel painting, but technically alien to some of the Italian sources influential in the style.

27

28

29

30

31

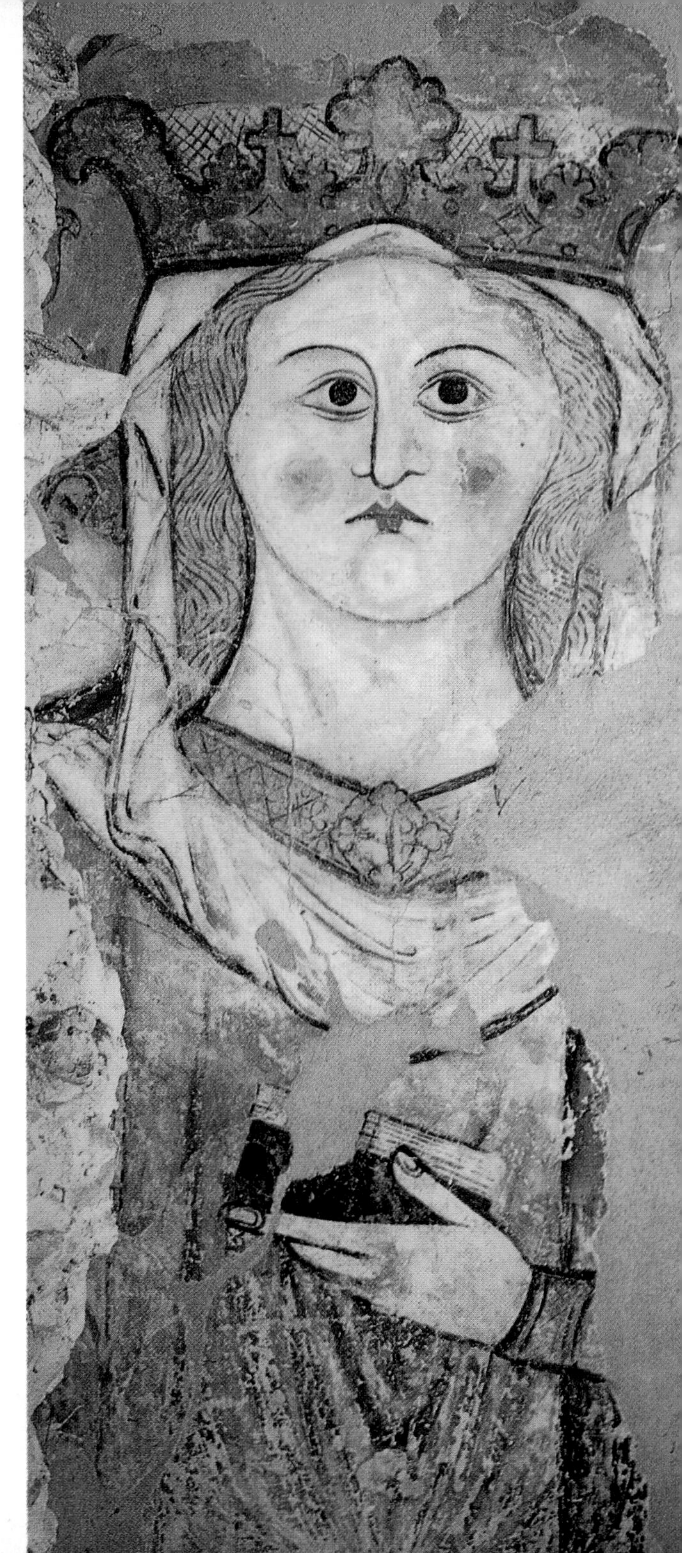

*Right* St Faith in the refectory of the Priory of Horsham St Faith, Norfolk, *c.* 1260, a magnificently well-preserved example of full-colour Gothic *secco* wall painting.

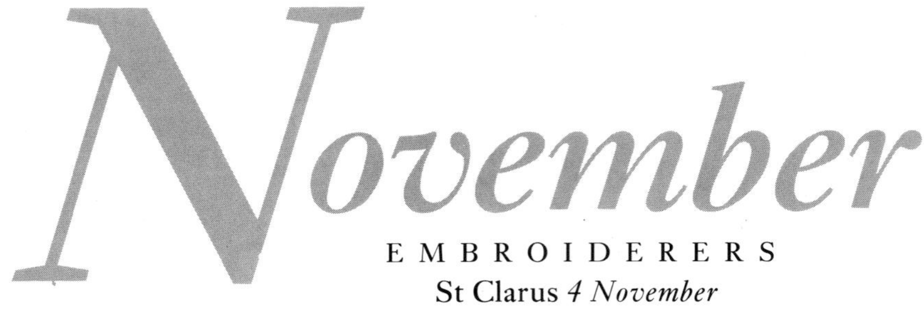

# November

EMBROIDERERS
St Clarus *4 November*

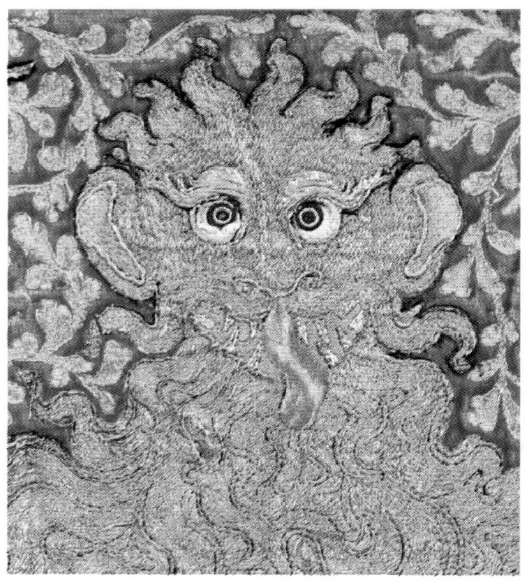

EMBROIDERY was a craft suitable for noble women and queens were often accredited with great skill in it. William of Malmesbury recorded that Queen Edith, wife of Edward the Confessor (1042–66), embroidered with her own hands the robes worn by the King at festivals. The equipment needed for embroidery was simple but the materials, the silk ground and the silver and gold thread, were often expensive. While simple embroideries could have been carried out by a single person, larger objects such as copes or altar pieces would have been the product of a workshop. The names of some of the ladies who supplied King Henry III of England (1216–72) with chasubles and other ecclesiastical embroidery are known. Mabel of Bury St Edmunds is mentioned most frequently and in 1256 we know that the King gave her a gift of cloth lined with rabbit fur as a reward for her long service.

Royal accounts often give us an insight into the nature of the workforce, the range of skills employed and the balance of men to women. For instance, in 1330, the making of the three counterpanes for the churching ceremonials of Queen Philippa, wife of Edward III, required 112 people, headed by two artist designers. There were 70 men earning 4d per day and 42 women earning 3d per day while the artist/designers earned 8d and 6d per day respectively, making a grand total of £60.17.6d.

A variety of techniques were employed in medieval embroidery, such as appliqué (stitching cloth pieces to a contrasting ground), the use of outline and filling stitches, cross stitch and counted thread embroidery. Couching and underside couching were techniques also widely used, the latter demanding great skill and declining in the 15th century.

Embroidery was often enriched with pearls, semi-precious stones and gold and silver ornaments and the effect of such sumptuous work on the observer must have been considerable.

1

2

3

4

Fragment of heraldic embroidery showing two of the three leopards of England worked in surface-couched gold thread and coloured silks. This is believed to have been a horse-covering made for Edward III in 1330–40.

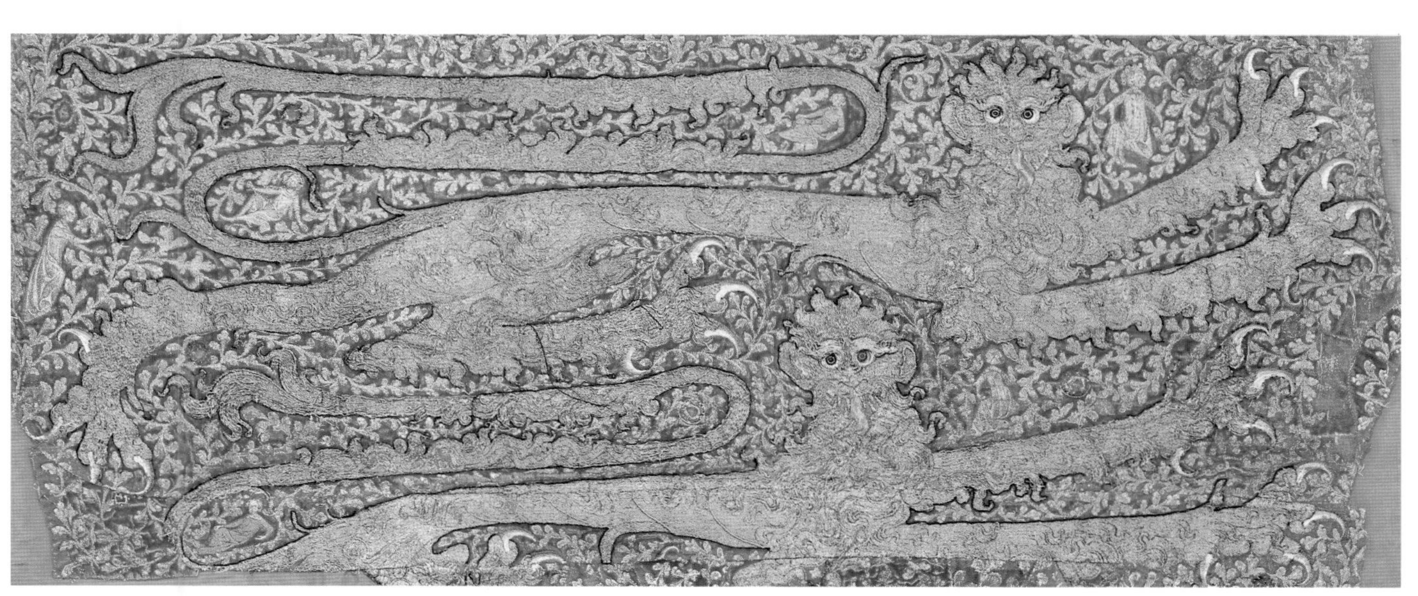

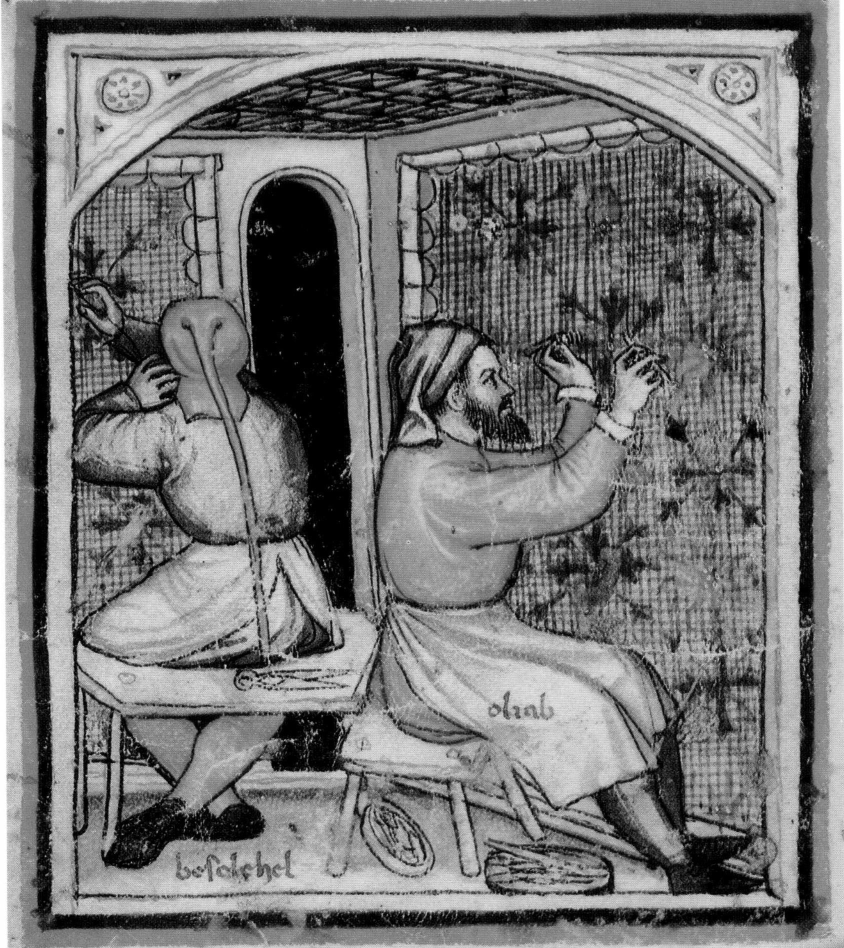


Jewish craftsmen at work on woven hangings stretched on a frame. From an Italian manuscript of *c.* 1400.

# November

5

6

7

8

The line above the picture records that Sir Geoffrey Luttrell (*Dns Galfridus Louterell*) caused this manuscript to be made (*me fieri fecit*). He is shown here on horseback being prepared for a tournament. His wife hands him his helm and standard, while his daughter-in-law approaches with the shield. It dates from between 1320 and 1340.

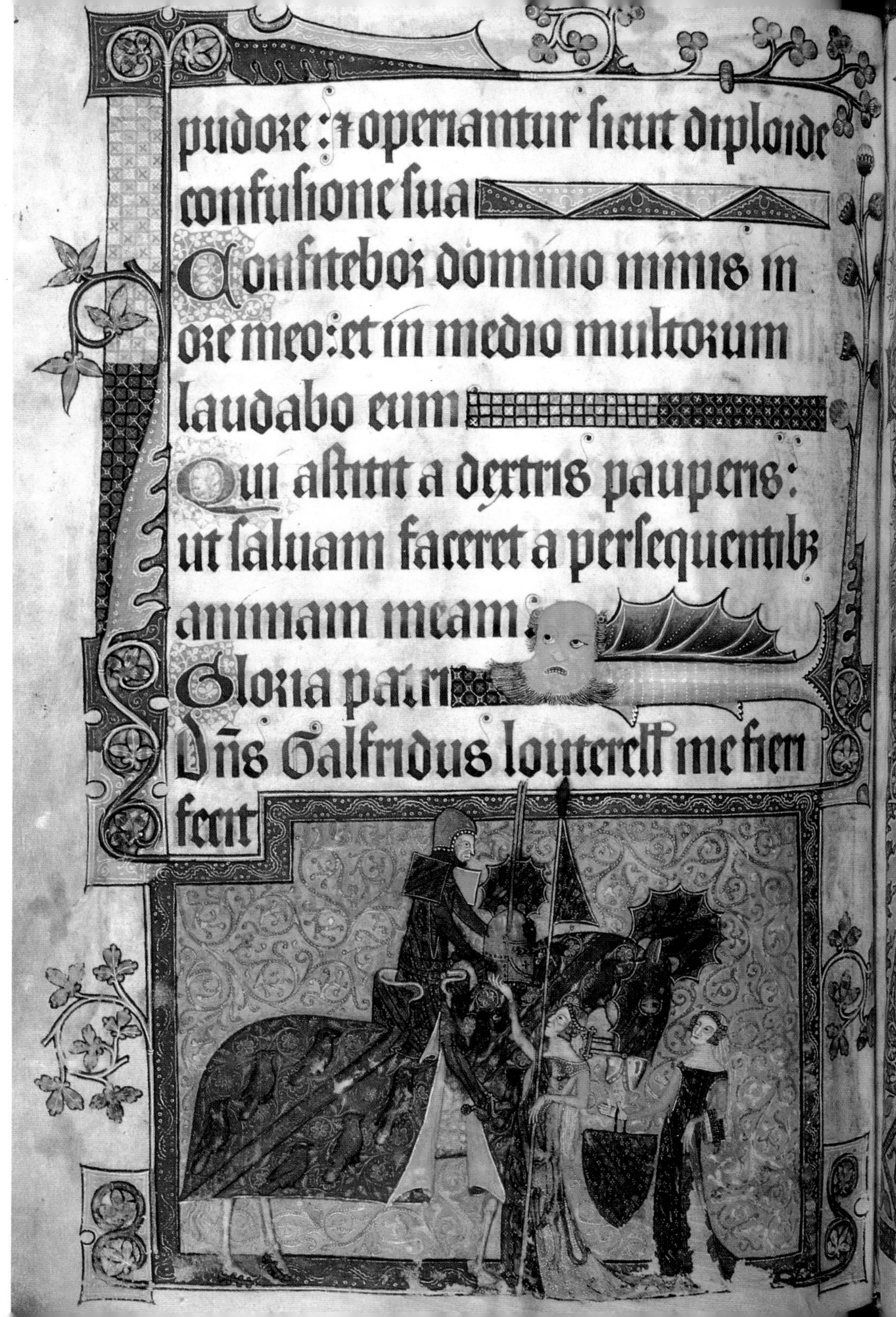

pudore: ⁊ operiantur sicut diploide
confusione sua
Confitebor domino nimis in
ore meo: et in medio multorum
laudabo eum
Qui astitit a dextris pauperis:
ut saluam faceret a persequentibꝫ
animam meam
Gloria patri
Dñs Galfridus louterell me fieri
fecit

# November

*Erly in a someristide*
*y sawe in London, as y wente,*
*A gentilwoman of chepe-side*
*workinge on a vestment.*

Late fifteenth-century poem showing that Cheapside in London was still a centre for embroiderers.

9

10

11

12

13

14

15

16

17

18

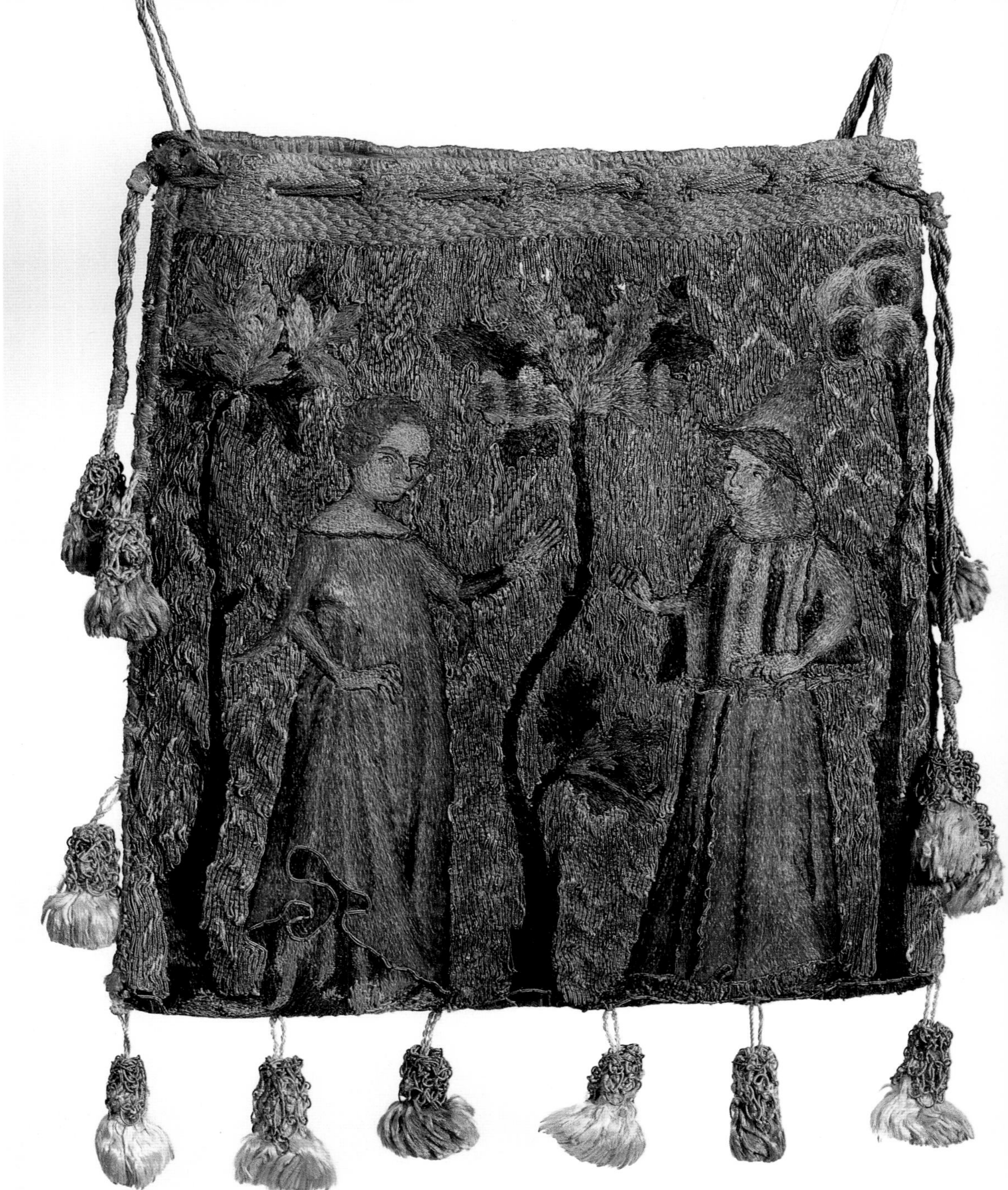

Purse (*aumonière*) depicting lovers, worked in Paris *c.* 1340. Linen embroidered in silk in split, chain, stem and knot stitches, the background of gold threads couched with red silk.

# November

19

20

21

22

23

24

25

26

27

28

In this palace bedchamber all the upholstery and hangings are decorated with the arms of France (fleurs-de-lis) and Bavaria (lozenges). The hangings are either stamped or embroidered with gold, the bed canopy and cover are almost certainly embroidered. Miniature from an early fifteenth-century French manuscript of the works of Christine de Pisan, showing the author presenting her book to Isabel of Bavaria, Queen of France, wife of Charles VI.

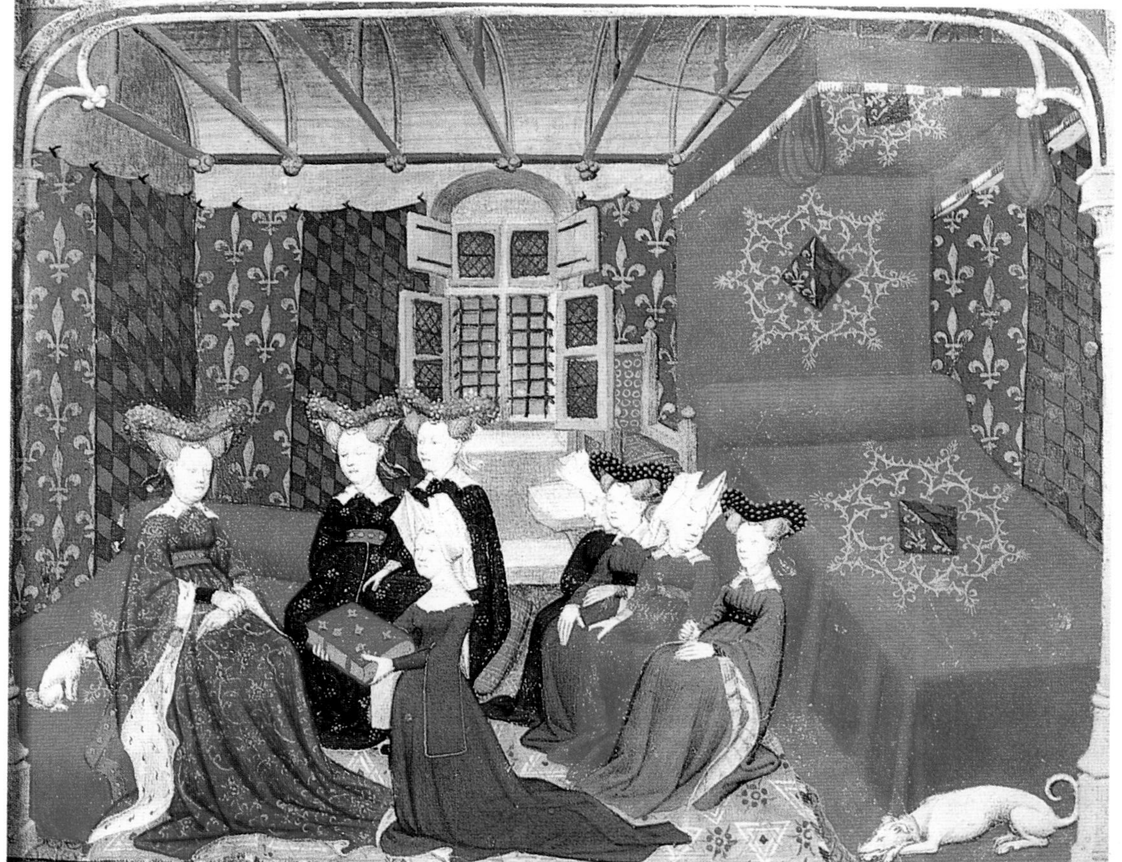

*29*

*30*

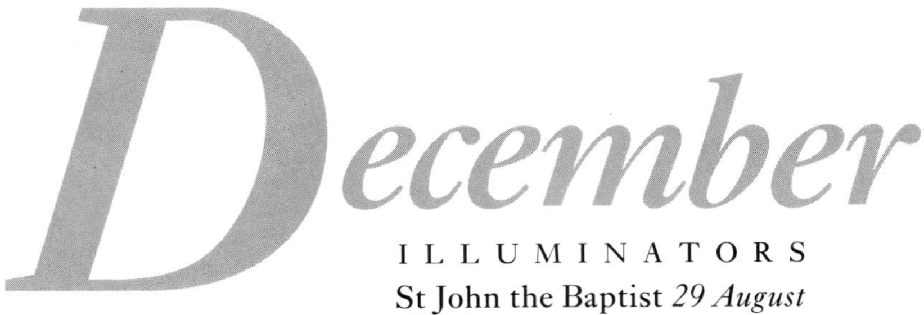


## ILLUMINATORS

St John the Baptist *29 August*

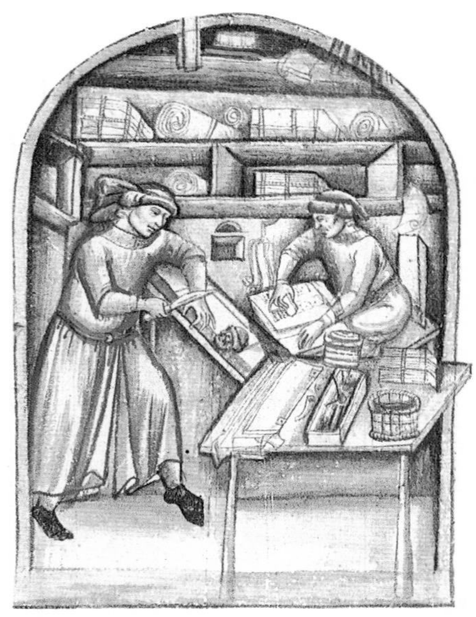

ILLUMINATED manuscripts with their rich and colourful borders and gilded pictures are one of the great delights of the Middle Ages. Each manuscript is different. Some have decoration on the first page, while others are decorated throughout the whole manuscript. Some have decorated line endings, while others have full borders filled with foliage amongst which rabbits, birds and grotesques clamber.

The very rare self portrait of Hugo Pictor, a late eleventh-century Norman monastic painter, shows a tonsured monk sitting holding a page down with a knife in his right hand. In contrast Simon Bening (a renowned sixteenth-century illuminator) was no monk. He married twice and had five legitimate children as well as an illegitimate daughter.

A wide range of colours was used by the medieval manuscript painter. Red was made from natural cinnabar or from such plants as brazil wood or madder. Blue was most commonly made from azurite or the seed of a plant called *crozophora*. The very best blue was made from lapis lazuli, which is only found naturally near Afghanistan. Other pigments included green from malachite or verdigris, yellow from saffron and white from white lead.

Most illuminators charged by the work rather than the time required to complete it. An account for a psalter decorated by Thomas Lympnour of Bury St Edmunds in 1467 indicates that full-page illuminations and half-page illustrations cost 4d each, small painted initials were 4d a hundred and capital letters a penny a hundred. This range of prices reflects the hierarchy of decoration.

An illuminated manuscript reflects light by its gold and silver. If gold leaf is to be applied, it must be put on before the colour, since the gold may stick to any pigment already laid, and the vigorous act of burnishing will smudge any painting. The shining of the burnished gold in manuscripts after so many hundred years is a tribute to the technical skill of the medieval illuminators.

*Left* A parchment-seller's shop illustrated in a fifteenth-century Italian chronicle. One man is trimming the sheets into rectangles and the other is rubbing them down with chalk in preparation for writing.

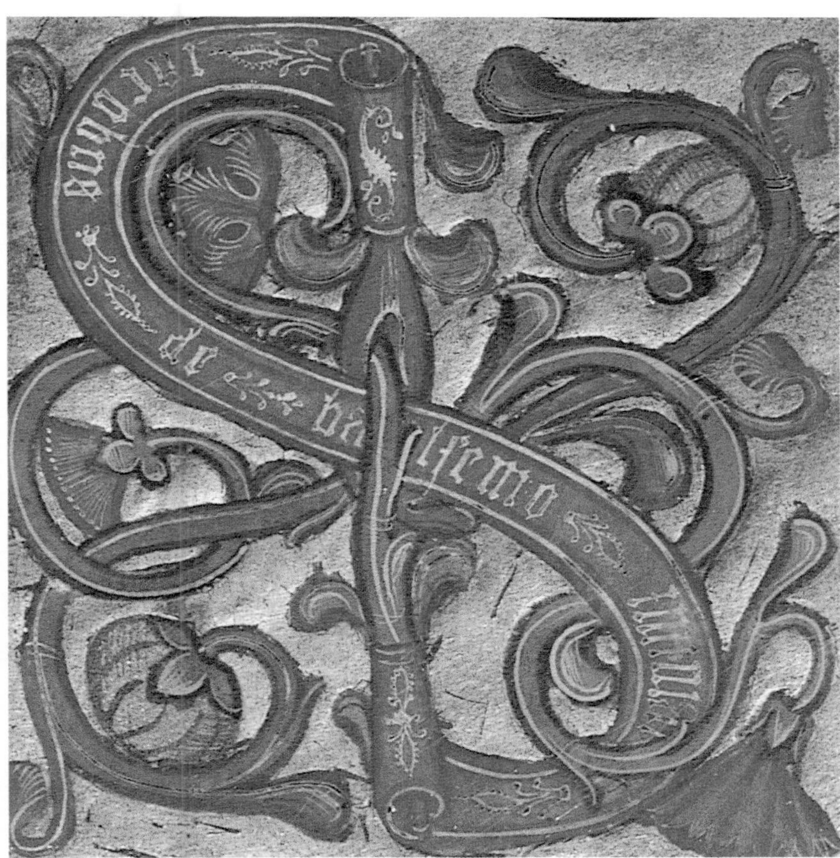

*Above* An illuminated initial signed in the scrollwork by the illuminator Jacopa da Balsemo (*c.* 1425–*c.* 1503) of Bergamo. Signed manuscript illumination is very uncommon.

*1*

*2*

*3*

*4*

*5*

# December

6

7

8

9

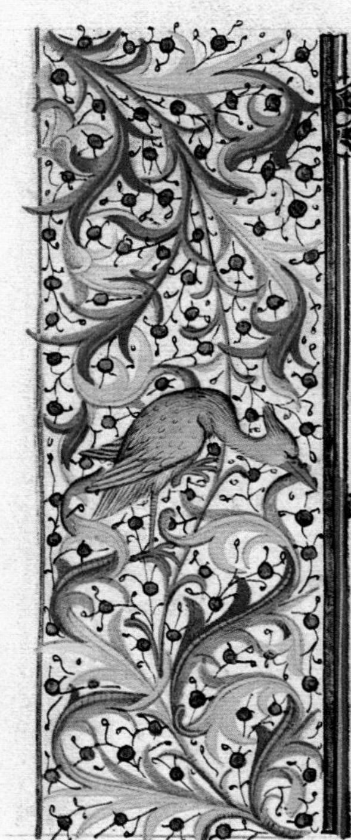

uit me.
Domine libera aiam meã
a labijs iniquis et a lingua
dolosa. Quid detur tibi aut
quid apponatur tibi ad lin
guam dolosam.
Sagitte potentis acute
cum carbonib; desolatoriis
Heu michi quia incolatus
meus, plongatus est habita
ui cum habitantib; cedar
multũ incola fuit aĩa mea
Cum hiis qui oderũt pacẽ
eram pacificus cum loquebar
illis impugnabãt me gratis

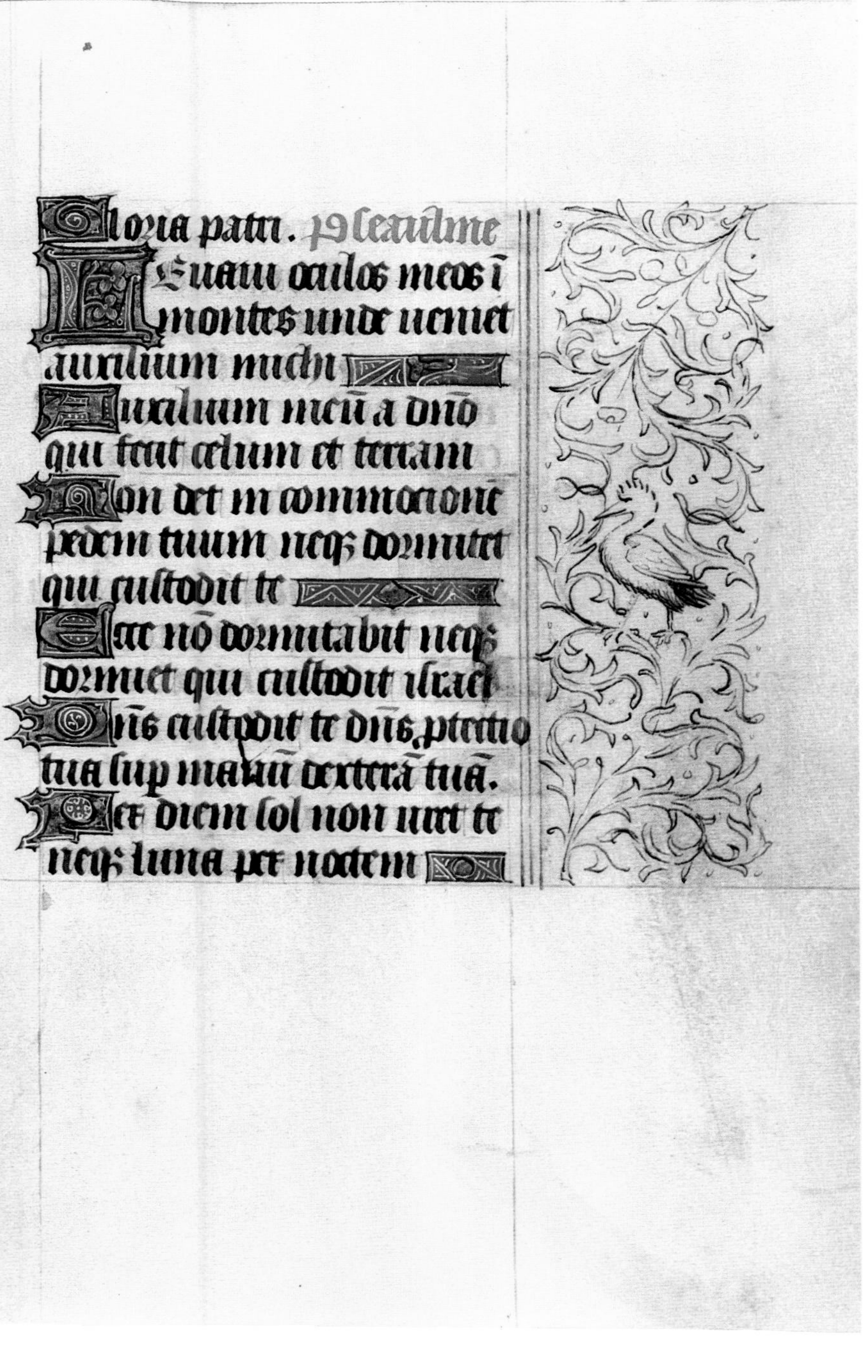

*10*

---

*11*

---

*12*

---

*13*

---

An opening from a partially-completed French Book of Hours. The border on the left is finished, but that on the right shows the preliminary sketch and the crisping-up in ink before the application of colour.

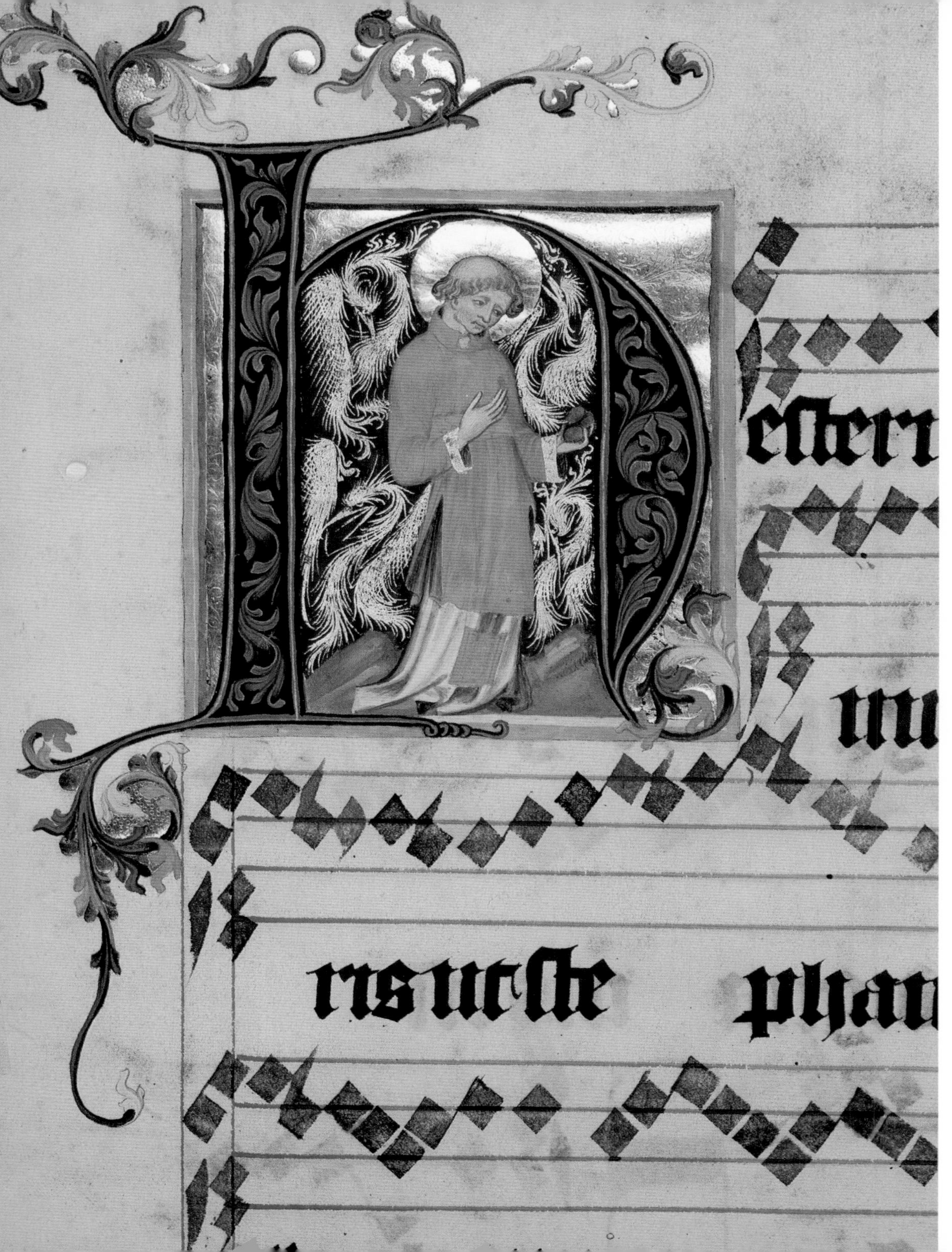

Two types of gold appear on this miniature of St Stephen from a choirbook illuminated in Prague *c.* 1405. The background of frenzied cockatrices behind the saint is painted with liquid or 'shell' gold, applied probably with a pen. But the halo and the surround are of burnished gold, applied as leaf laid over raised gesso. This has been not only burnished to a high finish, but also stamped on top with delicate patterns.

# December

14

15

16

17

18

19

20

21

22

23

*We, who are a light to faithful souls everywhere, fall prey to painters knowing nought of letters, and are entrusted to goldsmiths to become, as though we were not sacred vessels of wisdom, repositories of gold leaf.*

Complaint of the books in the *Philobiblon* written by Richard of Bury, bishop of Durham.

Saluator mundi salua
nos omnes sancta dei
genitrix uirgo semper maria
ora pro nobis. precibus quas

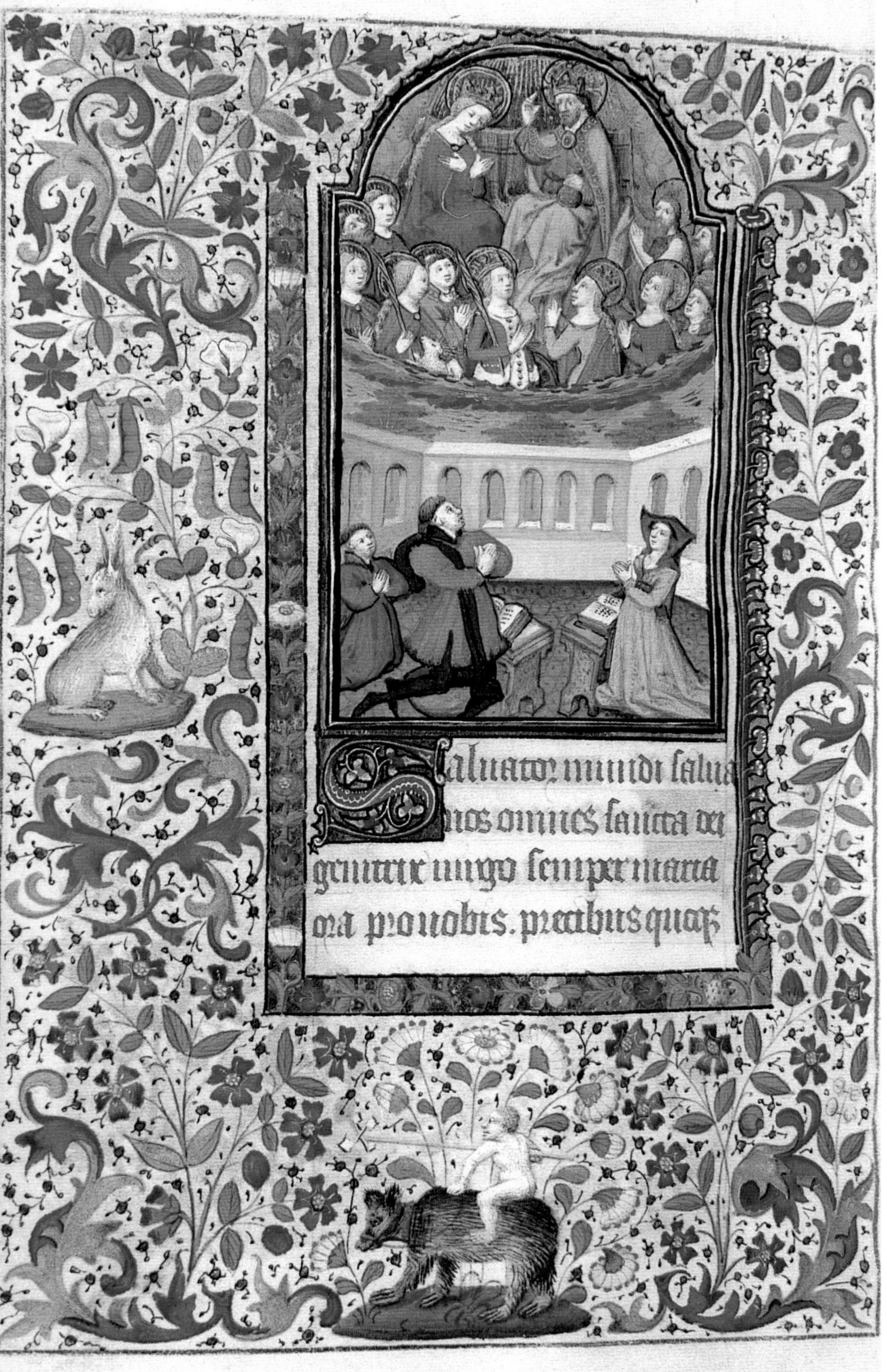

# December

24

25

26

*Right* The Devil tries to steal St John's inkpot and pencase to prevent him writing the Book of Revelation, *c.* 1480.

*Left* Illuminated page from a Parisian Book of Hours, *c.* 1440.

27

28

29

30

31

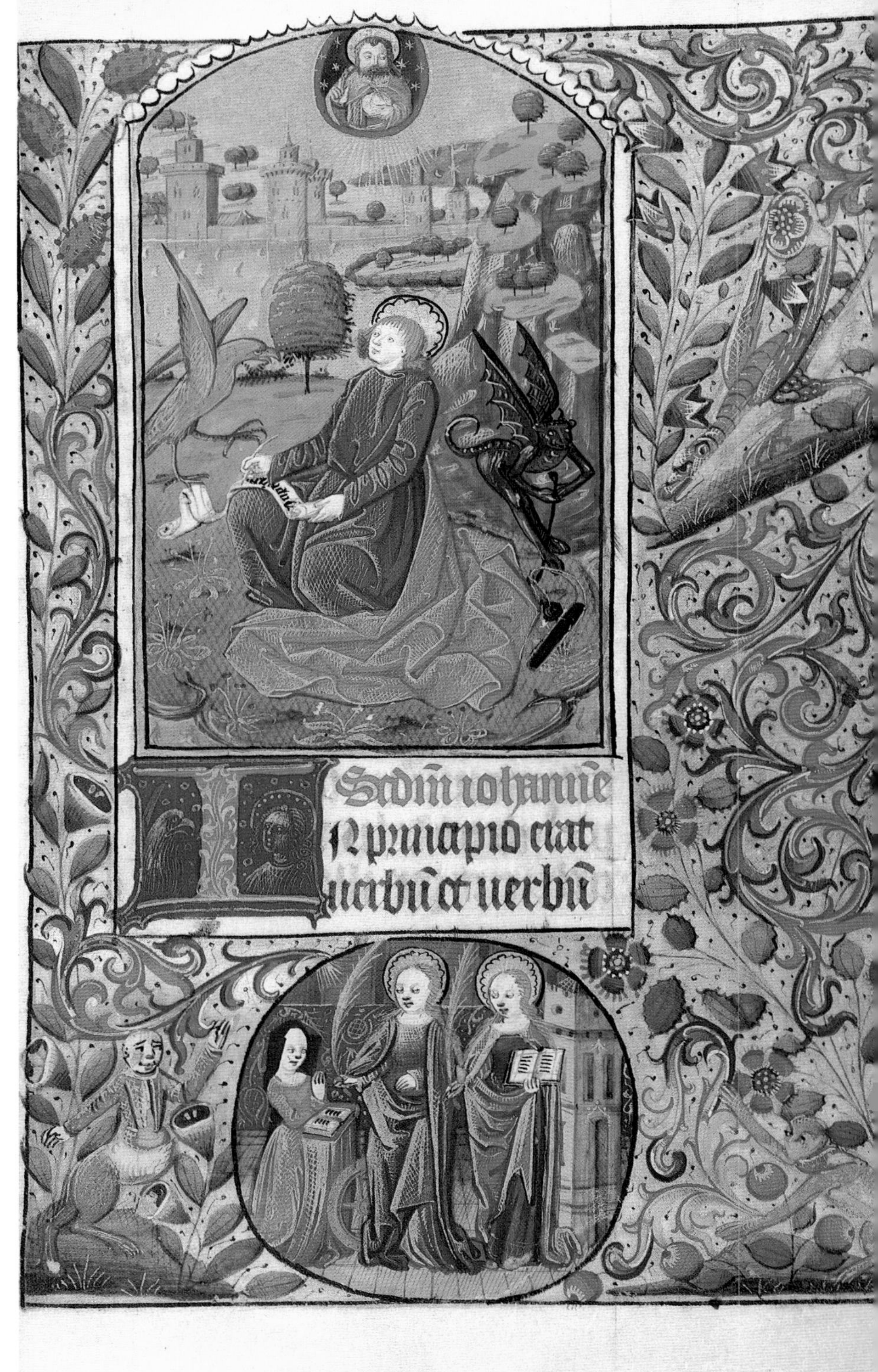

# Further Reading

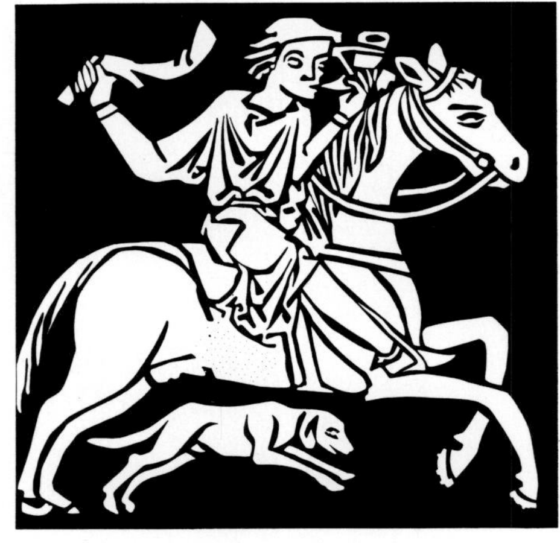

Designs on tiles in Westminster Abbey Chapter House.

Much of the material in this book has been drawn from the *Medieval Craftsmen* series published by British Museum Press in 1991 and 1992, and in North America by the University of Toronto Press.

*Armourers*
Matthias Pfaffenbichler

*Embroiderers*
Kay Staniland

*English Tilers*
Elizabeth Eames

*Glass-painters*
Sarah Brown David O'Connor

*Goldsmiths*
John Cherry

*Masons and Sculptors*
Nicola Coldstream

*Painters*
Paul Binski

*Scribes and Illuminators*
Christopher de Hamel

The recipe on page 74 and the illustrations from the Cooks' section are taken from *The Medieval Cookbook* by Maggie Black, published by the British Museum Press in 1992 and in North America by Thames and Hudson Inc.

Other titles of interest in this area are:

*Medieval Craftsmen*
John Harvey
Batsford, London 1975

*English Medieval Industries*
John Blair and Nigel Ramsay eds.
Hambledon Press, London 1991

*Church Bells of England*
H. B. Walters
Oxford University Press, 1912

*English Industries of the Middle Ages*
L. F. Salzman
Oxford University Press, 1927

*Trades and Crafts in Medieval Manuscripts*
P. Basing
British Library, London 1990

# Photo Acknowledgements

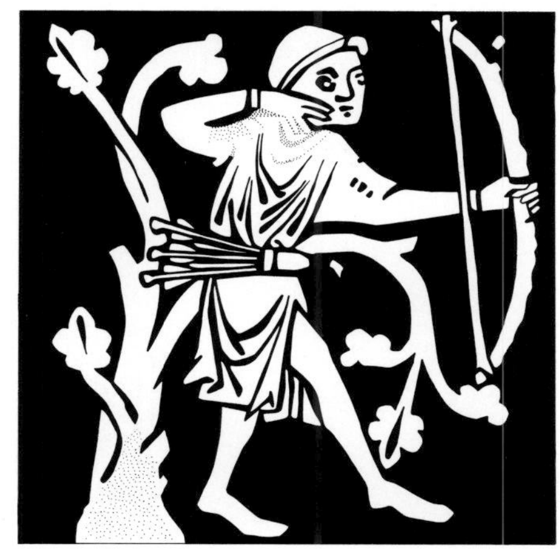

The author and publishers are grateful to the following people and institutions for permission to reproduce the illustrations listed below by page number.

Archives Municipales de Strasbourg (Photo: E. Laemmel): 7

Bayerisches Staatsbibliothek, Munich: 29

Bibliothèque Nationale, Paris: 20, 32, 38, 39, 43, 45, 64, 72, 86

Bodleian Library, Oxford: 56, 71, 104–5

City of Bristol Record Office: 70

The British Library, London: 1, 2, 24, 25, 41, 44–5, 57, 64, 75, 77, 78, 79, 87, 96, 97, 101

Trustees of the British Museum, London: 4, 10, 15, 48, 49, 52, 53, 55, 65, 67, 68, 81, 82, 83, 85, 92, 110, 111, 112

Musée de Cluny: 94, 95

Courtauld Institute, London (David Park): 93

Malcolm Crowthers, London: 88

The Dean and Chapter of Durham: 17

Germanisches Nationalmuseum, Nürnberg: 62

Sonia Halliday/Laura Lushington: 61

Kunsthistorischen Museums, Vienna: 46

Kunstmuseum, Berne: 50

The Board of the Trustees of the National Museums and Galleries on Merseyside (Liverpool Museum): 108

Museum für Kunst und Gewerbe, Hamburg: 99

Metropolitan Museum of Art, New York: 33

Österreichische Nationalbibliothek, Vienna: 30, 36, 89

Patrimonio Nacional, Madrid: 90–1

Pierpont Morgan Library, New York: 26

Pitkin Pictorial, Andover: 34

Real Armeria, Madrid: 40

Royal Library, Copenhagen: 16

St John's College, Cambridge: 19

Sothebys: 6, 18, 106, 109

Stoneyhurst College, Lancs: 13

Universitätsbibliothek, Heidelberg: 47

University Library, Bologna: 102

Dean and Chapter of Westminster: 22

Dean and Chapter of York: 9, 58, 63

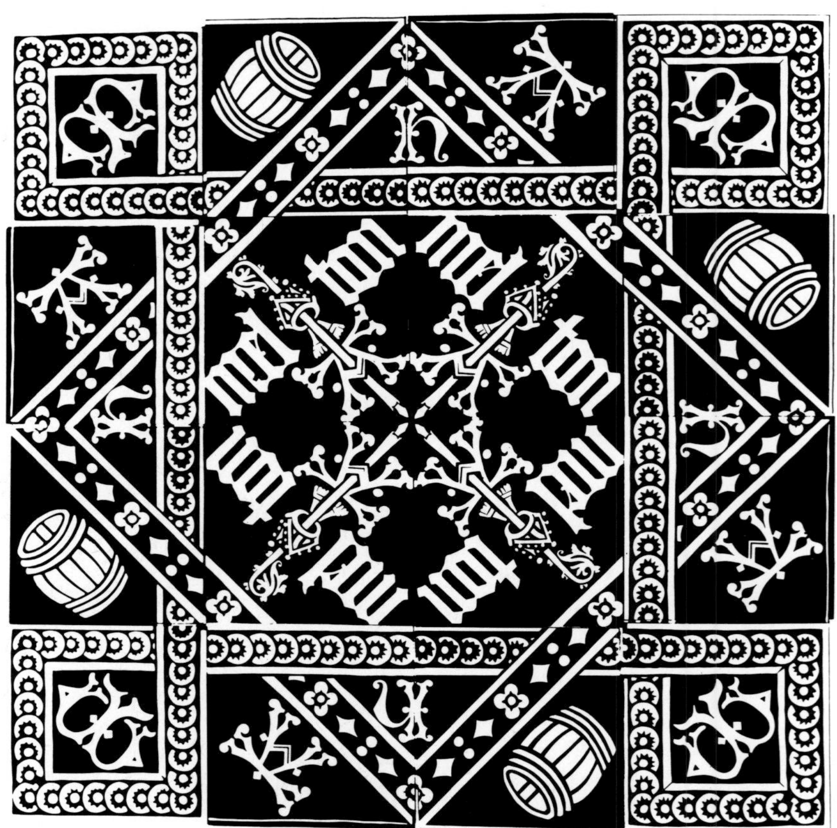

A sixteen-tile design on tiles from Hailes Abbey, Gloucestershire.